Counseling in Communication Disorders

Facilitating the Therapeutic Relationship

Counseling in Communication Disorders

Facilitating the Therapeutic Relationship

Cyndi Stein-Rubin, MS, CCC, TSSLD-SLP,
CTA Certified Coach
Retired Lecturer and Clinical Supervisor
Department of Speech, Language, and Hearing
Department
Brooklyn College of the City University of New York
Brooklyn, New York

Beryl T. Adler, MS, CCC, TSSH-SLP
Adler, Molly, Gurland, LLC
Adjunct Lecturer
Brooklyn College of the City University of New York
Brooklyn, New York

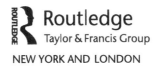

Routledge
Taylor & Francis Group

NEW YORK AND LONDON

Cyndi Stein-Rubin and Beryl T. Adler have no financial or proprietary interest in the materials presented herein.

Counseling in Communication Disorders: Facilitating the Therapeutic Relationship includes ancillary materials specifically available for faculty use. Included are Test Bank Questions, an Instructor's Manual. Please visit www.routledge.com/9781630912710

First published in 2017 by SLACK Incorporated

Published in 2024 by Routledge
605 Third Avenue, New York, NY 10158

and by Routledge
4 Park Square, Milton Park, Abingdon, Oxon, OX14 4RN

Routledge is an imprint of the Taylor & Francis Group, an informa business

© 2017 Taylor & Francis Group

Library of Congress Cataloging-in-Publication Data
Names: Stein-Rubin, Cyndi, author. | Adler, Beryl T., 1944- author.
Title: Counseling in communication disorders : facilitating the therapeutic
  relationship / Cyndi Stein-Rubin, Beryl T. Adler.
Description: Thorofare, NJ : SLACK Incorporated, [2017] | Includes
  bibliographical references and index.
Identifiers: LCCN 2016034257 (print) | ISBN
  9781630912710 (alk. paper)
Subjects: | MESH: Communication Disorders--therapy | Counseling--methods |
  Professional-Patient Relations
Classification: LCC RC423 (print) | NLM WL 340.2 | DDC
  616.85/506--dc23
LC record available at https://lccn.loc.gov/2016034257

ISBN: 9781630912710 (pbk)
ISBN: 9781003523352 (ebk)

DOI: 10.4324/9781003523352

DEDICATION

This book is dedicated to the people who have shaped who I have become—my precious family and the countless clients, families, and students who I have coached, treated, taught, supervised, and mentored over the past 33 years.

Cyndi Stein-Rubin, MS, CCC, TSSLD-SLP, CTA Certified Coach

To Dara, Bradley, Lauren, Emily, Rebecca, and Zachary.

To all of my family and extended family, and to all those families I have worked with through the many years of my career. You have all inspired me.

Beryl T. Adler, MS, CCC, TSSH-SLP

CONTENTS

ACKNOWLEDGMENTS

I want to express my deep gratitude to my loving and devoted husband, Jeff, for his patience, support, and sense of humor—invaluable attributes in helping bring our work to fruition. I also want to acknowledge my beautiful sons, daughters-in-law, and grandchildren for their love, support, and inspiration. Thank you very much to Sarah Golda Ackerman-Westreich and Dana Levine-Buccelato for their substantive contributions and feedback. I would also like to acknowledge my wonderful parents, Ann and Raanan Wertheim (may my Dad rest in peace) for instilling in us the values of education, developing a professional career, and for all the sacrifices they made along the way. To my dear in-laws, Mimi and Howard Rubin, who have been a constant source of support and interest in my work. I will always be grateful and delighted by their enthusiasm and curiosity. Finally, I'd like to thank my illustrious co-writer, Beryl Adler, who is a joy to work with and also a role model for supportive authentic communication and teamwork. I looked forward to each time we work together.

Cyndi Stein-Rubin, MS, CCC, TSSLD-SLP, CTA Certified Coach

There are always so many people to acknowledge with gratitude and deep appreciation for their contributions to my life…the list begins with my mother, Sharon Modell, who always believed in listening and hearing the voice of a child. My children, Dara and Bradley, taught me so much about parenting and moving beyond what we think our children need. I have been able to share this knowledge with Lauren and my grandchildren.

I have had the opportunity to create a wonderful practice in this extraordinary profession with Gail Gurland and Leda Molly. We are fortunate to have served as coaches to each other throughout the years.

The many students, therapists, clients, families, and office staff that I have been honored to work with have provided me with experiences that will last a lifetime. Everyday continues to be filled with something new, exciting, and challenging to learn.

This book would have not happened without the determination, encouragement, and vision of my co-author, Cyndi Stein-Rubin. Cyndi truly believed that this was a project for us to complete together. It has been a rich and rewarding learning experience. Our book represents our process.

Lastly, I will always be indebted and grateful to Professor Gail Gurland, who called one day in 1984 and asked me to teach the Therapeutic Relationships Course at Brooklyn College. She provided the opportunity for me to develop this material. She truly continues to support and inspire all my life's endeavors.

Thank you all.

Beryl T. Adler, MS, CCC, TSSH-SLP

ABOUT THE AUTHORS

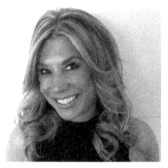

Cyndi Stein-Rubin, MS, CCC, TSSLD-SLP, CTA Certified Coach is a retired full-time faculty member, lecturer, and clinical supervisor in the Department of Speech, Language and Hearing Department Brooklyn College of the City University of New York (CUNY). She is a certified speech-language pathologist, professional life coach, and specialist in the field of human development. Mrs. Stein-Rubin the recipient of the 2009 college-wide Award for Excellence in Teaching and has served on the committee, for the past 4 years to select future award winners. Her area of expertise is in coaching and counseling students, clients, and families in the area of communication disorders, and her private practice focuses primarily on adults with disorders of fluency and voice. Cyndi Stein-Rubin delivers interactive and experiential workshops and presentations, drawing from fields such as psychology, counseling, and leadership. She lectures at universities, in the community, as well as internationally. Cyndi Stein-Rubin, is the first author of a co-authored textbook, *A Guide to Clinical Assessment and Professional Report Writing in Speech-Language Pathology* (Cengage Learning, 2012). *Counseling in Communication Disorders: Facilitating the Therapeutic Relationship* is her second book, co-authored by Beryl Adler.

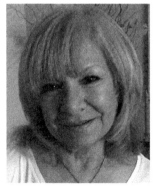

Beryl T. Adler, MS, CCC, TSSH-SLP has been a practicing speech-language pathologist for over 40 years, with extensive experience in language, articulation, fluency, and voice disorders. She received her master of science degree from Brooklyn College in New York in 1969. During her career, she has worked as a Clinical Supervisor and Instructor at the Brooklyn College Speech and Hearing Center and as an Adjunct Lecturer at Westbury Community College in New York and Brooklyn College, where she has taught a variety of courses in speech and language disorders. She founded Beryl Adler and Associates, a private practice in Brooklyn, in 1978. By 1984 she joined with Leda Molly and Gail Gurland to form Adler, Molly, Gurland with offices in Brooklyn and Manhattan. Ms. Adler's expertise and applied research in counseling families led to the development of a graduate course on the therapeutic relationship in communication disorders, which she has taught at Brooklyn College since 1988. Ms. Adler has presented workshops for parents, teachers, therapists, and supervisors throughout New York City. In 2012, she received the Speech-Language-Hearing Graduate Student Organization Distinguished Alumna Award for her contribution to the graduate students at Brooklyn College.

INTRODUCTION

As we look back on close to 40 years as speech-language pathologist, we recognize how extraordinary our respective journeys have been.[1] Professionally, we have faced countless challenges with thousands of adults, children, and families. We have faced personal challenges within our own families and within ourselves as well. We have spent many years in school and in the field learning a variety of skills from masters and mentors. We have dedicated hours upon hours to teaching classes, advising, supervising clinicians, diagnosing, and administering direct therapy. The courses we have taught and the many hours we have logged with patients have been eye-opening, exciting, inspiring, and, at times, difficult.

To do our work effectively, we have had to learn beyond the information contained in textbooks and theories—about life, listening, resilience, strength, and the human condition. To become models for our students and clients, we have committed ourselves to ongoing personal growth and transformation. As we look not only back, but also ahead, we marvel at our path and feel astonished and grateful.

Over time, to become a resource for others, we have expanded our knowledge base beyond the content of our profession. We have learned the value of partnership in all forms, both professionally and personally, and that each person we meet brings us new lessons. We have learned the meaning of compromise and negotiation. We have each attempted to find educational value in our daily experiences and to look for potential and possibilities in everyone and everything. We have also learned we need to listen deeply and we need not have all the answers; what's most important is to ask more powerful and different kinds of questions. Through collaboration and partnership we have learned to live our lives more consciously (Geller, 2002). Finally, we have learned that despite our knowledge and experience, we always have more to learn. We are and have always been excited and energized about learning and about how our students, clients, and their families learn and grow. Growth has intrinsic rewards.

DEVELOPMENT OF OUR TEXTBOOK

We had a wonderful opportunity to combine our experiences, ideas, life lessons, and roles as diagnosticians, therapists, and instructors to co-write a counseling chapter for *A Guide to Clinical Assessment and Professional Report Writing for the Speech-Language Pathologist* (Stein-Rubin & Adler, 2012). After the book's publication, we were encouraged by colleagues to write our own book focusing on the personal development of the clinician as it relates to facilitating the counseling process and the therapeutic relationship.

Several counseling and interviewing textbooks and articles have been written for the speech-language pathologist and the audiologist. These works are comprehensive, well written, and valuable. Many of them explain counseling approaches theoretically and offer a number of suggestions for the counselor. What's missing, however, is a program or textbook that includes the most crucial elements in counseling efficacy: the personal development and mindfulness of the speech-language pathologist and audiologist in the therapeutic relationship (Ben-Shahar, 2010; Geller, 2002; Geller & Foley, 2009; Norcross, 2005; Reivich & Shatté, 2002; Rogers, 1951; Seligman, 2002).

---

[1]Please note that throughout this book, when we relate personal and clinical anecdotes, we use the initials CSR for Cyndi Stein-Rubin and BTA for Beryl T. Adler. In addition, we alternate between the use of he and she in case examples and other uses of singular personal pronouns.

Although our book discusses a variety of theories, it is also predicated on the idea that counseling, facilitating, and coaching are hands-on experiential processes. Listening to explanations and comparing theories won't suffice when it comes to developing the self-awareness and insight that the coaching process demands. *Counseling in Communication Disorders: Facilitating the Therapeutic Relationship* is an experiential, pragmatic, and interactive book.

The content of this book is based on a combination of disciplines, including humanistic counseling, positive psychology, solution-focused brief therapy, cognitive behavioral therapy, narrative therapy, motivational psychology, neurolinguistic programming, mindfulness training, and the Co-Active Coaching model. We have drawn from the literature in fields such as speech-language pathology, psychology, counseling, medicine, nursing, education, business, and leadership. In addition, we have incorporated information from workshops through Landmark Education and the Omega Health Institute. When individuals learn theory and develop skills by practicing and applying these approaches, there is an impact on all human relationships—professional and personal. Furthermore, as individuals learn new and different ways of interacting, there is an opportunity to practice with family members and friends in real time (Andrews, 2004).

Each chapter of our book introduces a new conversation, which includes case histories, clinical examples, and reflective and interactive exercises. It is of utmost importance for the reader to complete these exercises, throughout and at the conclusion of each chapter, in writing. Writing down reflective thoughts will help embed these concepts in one's memory and psyche. Do not underestimate the "power of the almighty pen."

Instructor's materials are offered at www.efacultylounge.com including a syllabus and sample final examination.

REFERENCES

Andrews, M. A. (2004). Clinical issues: Counseling techniques for speech-language pathologists. *SIG 1 Perspectives on Language, Learning, and Education, 11*(1), 3–8.

Ben-Shahar, T. (2010). *Foundations of positive psychology* [PowerPoint slides]. Retrieved from www.slideshare.net/dadalaolang/1504-01intro?ref=http://positivepsychologyprogram.com/harvard-positive-psychology-course.

Geller, E. (2002). A reflective model of supervision in speech-language pathology: Process and practice. *The Clinical Supervisor, 20*(2), 191–200.

Geller, E., & Foley, F. (2009). Broadening the "ports of entry" for speech-language pathologists: A relational and reflective model for clinical supervision. *American Journal of Speech-Language Pathology, 18*(1), 22–41.

Norcross, J. C. (2005). The psychotherapist's own psychotherapy: Educating and developing psychologists. *American Psychologist, 60*(8), 840–850.

Reivich, K., & Shatté, A. (2002). *The resilience factor: 7 essential skills for overcoming life's inevitable obstacles.* New York, NY: Broadway Books.

Rogers, C. R. (1951). *Client-centered therapy: Its current practice, implications and theory.* Boston, MA: Houghton Mifflin.

Seligman, M. E. (2002). *Authentic happiness: Using the new positive psychology to realize your potential for lasting fulfillment.* New York, NY: Free Press.

Stein-Rubin, C., & Adler, B. T. (2012). Counseling and the diagnostic interview for the speech-language pathologist. In C. Stein-Rubin & R. Fabus (Eds.), *A guide to clinical assessment and professional report writing in speech-language pathology* (pp. 9–40). Clifton Park, NY: Delmar Cengage Learning.

I

Powerful Perspectives

To do our work effectively, we have found that knowing ourselves goes hand-in-hand with the three powerful perspectives: counselor congruence, permission to be human, and client as expert. When we develop the frame of mind that includes these perspectives, and when we incorporate them into our communication, we are more sensitive, authentic, and motivating for our clients. These perspectives encourage us to become self-aware and to self-manage our emotions to more effectively help our clients achieve their goals.

We must be ready and willing to adopt these attitudes, just as our clients and their families must be ready and willing for intervention and the therapeutic process. According to Stein-Rubin and Adler (2012), "Readiness is timed when the client is primed."

REFERENCE

Stein-Rubin, C., & Adler, B. T. (2012). Counseling and the diagnostic interview for the speech-language pathologist. In C. Stein-Rubin & R. Fabus (Eds.), *A guide to clinical assessment and professional report writing in speech-language pathology* (pp. 9–40). Clifton Park, NY: Delmar Cengage Learning.

1

Know Yourself

We cannot become who we need to be by staying the same.

—Max Dupree, 2004

LEARNER OUTCOMES

After reading this chapter, the reader will be able to:

1. Discuss the importance of developing the self for the therapeutic relationship.

2. Explain the role of narratives in the clinical realm.

3. Describe the importance of counseling in our profession and our clinical role in counseling.

THE IMPORTANCE OF DEVELOPING OURSELVES FOR THE THERAPEUTIC RELATIONSHIP

Research in the field of psychotherapy has shown that the quality of the therapeutic alliance, or relationship, is the most significant predictor of treatment success (Friedman, 1969; Geller, 2002; Geller & Foley, 2009; Horvath & Laborsky, 1993; Krupnick et al., 1996; Marziali & Alexander, 1991; Safran & Muran, 2000). In our field, there is a paucity of information in the literature on developing the *self* to become the kind of person who facilitates powerful therapeutic relationships.

Through the years, we have found it is of paramount importance to employ various forms of listening and verbal expression to broaden our perspectives and see beyond our expectations. We have had to examine our own resistance to change and learn to accept our clients' agendas. We have also had to look closely at our need to be "right," our own flexibility, our willingness to compromise, and our personal relationships with our own

Stein-Rubin, C., & Adler, B. T. *Counseling in Communication Disorders: Facilitating the Therapeutic Rehabilitation* (pp 3-8). © 2017 Taylor & Francis Group.

vulnerabilities and limitations. As such, we may become a source to facilitate a powerful therapeutic relationship.

We have further witnessed how new clinicians become confused, disillusioned, frustrated, and burned out when clients and clients' families neglect to follow through on their professional recommendations. Often, these recommendations are met with resistance. Through our conversations with new clinicians, we often learn that our supervisees do not know themselves and the human condition well enough to mitigate resistance and to manage it if it occurs.

Counseling Defined

Counseling in communication disorders may be defined as an applied social science and an interpersonal relationship that involves helping clients and their families understand and prevent the possibility of further deterioration of their communication (Flasher & Fogel, 2012). Furthermore, counseling involves empowering clients to cope with and adjust to the challenges of a speech-language, hearing, or swallowing disorder (Zebrowski & Schum, 1993).

There is both a science and an art to counseling. The science part of counseling may be thought of as theoretical, where we familiarize ourselves with the basic theoretical approaches of counseling, which is necessary given the scope of our practice (Flasher & Fogel, 2011). This scientific aspect of counseling reflects a more traditional medical model, which focuses on disseminating content, providing diagnostic results, clarifying information, recommending treatment procedures, and dispensing advice. In this model, the clinician assumes the role of the expert or teacher; for example, the clinician may provide advice to parents on how to talk to a child who stutters by reducing speech pressure (Zebrowski & Schum, 1993). Geller and Foley (2009) refer to this model as an *outside-in approach*.

Yet according to DiLollo (2010), many health-related professions have begun to question the effectiveness of the exclusive use of the medical model in achieving client independence and maximizing therapeutic results. Thus, health professions have been moving toward a more person-centered approach based on Carl Rogers' humanistic therapy.

The art form of counseling, which is more person-centered and focuses on the emotions and feelings of the client or family members (or both), depends on the empathy of the counselor, his knowledge and expertise in demonstrating these skills, and the awareness that client readiness and timing are essential. An empathic counselor would be concerned with the client's and family members' attitudes, emotions, and struggles surrounding the disorder and how to access, explore, and reframe what may be habitual negative thinking patterns (Riley, 2002). The art aspect and/or person-centered approach are also focused on the client–family–clinician relationship, placing the client in the center of the relationship and viewing him as an expert who has a shared power with the clinician and is an *inside-out approach* (Geller & Foley, 2009). Therefore, to provide optimal services for their clients and families, clinicians must have knowledge about the disorders they will encounter and be educated in both aspects of counseling.

Furthermore, it has been our clinical experience, and it has also been noted in the literature, that clinicians training to practice the transformative art of counseling must work on *self* before working on *other*. Until counselors develop a relationship with themselves, they will be unable to approach clients with authenticity. It has been shown that clinicians often prefer to avoid emotional counseling moments, yet it is nonetheless essential that they be mindful of these inner thoughts and beliefs to cultivate relationships with their clients (Bradshaw & Gregory, 2014).

WE ALL HAVE A STORY TO TELL

Across cultures, languages, religions, genders, and ages, everyone has a story to tell. Our stories help clarify the events and circumstances of our lives. They reveal our emotions, personalities, and sense of humor. Telling stories helps forge bonds in our relationships, maintain our histories and our cultures. In a piece on the *Today* show Bob Dotson (2015), the great American storyteller and news correspondent, commented that, "The shortest distance between two people is their story." Through story, we teach our children good values and life lessons, and validate their emotions. An important part of our role as speech-language pathologists is to help our clients tell their stories. Many of their stories reflect the impact of their challenges on themselves and on their lives. These narratives also shed light on their unique nature and how we may be of the most help to them (Page, 2015).

Dr. Oliver Sacks used his patients' narratives as a way to help them medically and as a teaching tool. At first, this was a very different and unaccepted way to address medicine, which had become data driven. Eventually, Dr. Sacks' focus revolutionized the way that physicians approached the case history. This was a different way to approach medicine, and over time, his use of narratives became understood and accepted (Silberman, 2015).

As speech-language pathologists and audiologists, stories have a significant place in the diagnosis and intervention process. There are several articles in the psychological literature that discuss the importance of client narratives in the therapeutic process (Carpenter, Brockopp, & Andrykowski, 1999; Facione & Giancarlo, 1998; Morse & O'Brien, 1995; Pennebaker & Seagal, 1999).

Although storytelling is often cathartic and supportive for the person telling the story, it is important that the individual not get stuck in his narrative. Eventually, clients may need to alter their stories into more empowering ones to make the desired progress. We need to provide clients with the opportunity to recognize small gains and to discuss their achievements.

Clinician Stories and Teaching Moments

Clinicians also have stories specific to their own lives as well as stories specific to their clients. Instructors, clinical supervisors, clinicians, and public speakers use stories to illustrate a point. Most of our students have expressed that the stories we shared made the material more realistic for them, helped them to remember what they were learning, and inspired them to learn how to handle clinical interactions.

Clinicians must be able to distinguish their own stories from those of their clients' to maintain professional boundaries. Although as clinicians we must empathize with our clients' stories, it is crucial that we maintain objectivity. Refer to the section on judgment in Chapter 9 for information on self-management.

Throughout the book, we will be telling some of our own stories, the stories of some of our clients, and stories that we have heard from others. It is important to note that when relating clinical narratives, we must withhold the names of clients and family members in accordance with the Health Insurance Portability and Accountability Act.

DEFINING OUR PROFESSIONAL ROLE

Although we are not psychologists, it is crucial that we, as speech, language, and hearing clinicians, familiarize ourselves and become versed in counseling approaches that pertain to the communication disorders of our clients and their families. It is understandable if our clients or family members cry or otherwise express upset, disappointment, sadness, and anxiety. These are normal human emotions in response to a catastrophic or life-altering event and may occur as individuals struggle with a communication disorder (Bradshaw & Gregory, 2014; Luterman, 2008).

At the same time, we must also learn to distinguish when we may need to step back and to stay within our scope of practice. There are situations that may require us to offer a suggestion and recommend that professionals in other domains address certain aspects of our clients' cognitive, emotional, or physical states (Box 1-1).

Box 1-1

One morning a couple came to my (BTA) office complaining of the gentleman's vocal hoarseness. He had been referred for voice therapy by several ear, nose, and throat physicians. The gentleman was severely hoarse, required intervention, and surgery was not recommended. During the interview, the gentleman blamed his wife, who was in the waiting room, for his vocal stress and strain. When his wife entered the room, they argued, shouted, and constantly blamed each other. Through discussion, the couple came to the conclusion that nothing would help the gentleman's hoarseness, if they were to continue in this pattern.

We then discussed alternatives that might be helpful before initiating voice therapy, and I referred them to a marriage counselor. I spoke with them a year later, and the gentleman was doing much better. As their interpersonal communication improved, so did his voice.

We, as communication professionals, need to understand our scope of practice, skills, and limitations. There is a time to collaborate and refer to other professionals who are more skilled and trained for some of the situations we may encounter. When making recommendations to clients, it is helpful to preface these by saying, "May I offer a suggestion?" (Kimsey-House, Kimsey-House, Sandahl, & Whitworth, 2011). This question empowers clients, helps them to own their decision, and makes it more likely that they will follow through on the suggestions.

Conclusion

Although this book is focused on the therapeutic relationship among clinician, client, and family, we will also refer to additional alliances such as supervisor-supervisee, instructor–student, and parent–child. Furthermore, the lessons in this book are applicable to the general public and to everyday interactions. Our hope is that this textbook will inspire the reader to grow, expand his perspective about counseling, and deepen the therapeutic relationship. An essential ingredient for change is action, and thus we encourage the reader to engage with the material, take ownership of the work, and be fully present to the process.

It is important to note that if you are suffering from depression, an anxiety disorder, mood swings, obsessive thinking, addiction, or other disorders that interfere with your functioning or well-being, this book should not be used as a substitute for appropriate professional intervention.

References

Bradshaw, J., & Gregory, K. (2014). The other side of CCCs: Communication, counseling and clinicians. *The ASHA Leader.* Online only. doi:10.1044/leader.FTR4.19052014.np.

Carpenter, J. S., Brockopp, D. Y., & Andrykowski, M. A. (1999). Self-transformation as a factor in the self-esteem and well-being of breast cancer survivors. *Journal of Advanced Nursing, 29*(6), 1402–1411.

DiLollo, A. (2010). Business: The crisis of confidence in professional knowledge: Implications for clinical education in speech-language pathology. *Sig 11 Perspectives on Administration and Supervision, 20,* 85-91. doi:10.1044/aas20.3.85.

Dotson, B. (2015). 40 years of American story-telling: A veteran NBC News correspondent looks back. *Today.* Retrieved from www.today.com/news/40-years-american-storytelling-veteran-nbc-news-correspondent-looks-back-t51216

Dupree, M. (2004). *Leadership is an art.* New York, NY: Crown Publishing Group.

Facione, N. C., & Giancarlo, C. A. (1998). Narratives of breast symptom discovery and cancer diagnosis: Psychological risk for advanced cancer at diagnosis. *Cancer Nursing, 21*(6), 430–440.

Flasher, L., & Fogle, P. (2012). *Counseling skills for speech-language pathologists and audiologists.* Clifton Park, NY: Delmar Cengage Learning.

Friedman, L. (1969). Negotiating the therapeutic alliance: A relational treatment guide. *The International Journal of Psychoanalysis, 50*(2), 139–153.

Geller, E. (2002). A reflective model of supervision in speech-language pathology: Process and practice. *The Clinical Supervisor, 20*(2), 191–200.

Geller, E., & Foley, F. (2009). Broadening the "ports of entry" for speech-language pathologists: A relational and reflective model for clinical supervision. *American Journal of Speech-Language Pathology, 18*(1), 22–41.

Horvath, A. O., & Luborsky, F. (1993). The role of the therapeutic alliance in psychotherapy. *Journal of Consulting and Clinical Psychology, 61*(4), 561–573.

Kimsey-House, H., Kimsey-House, K., Sandahl, P., & Whitworth, L. (2011). *Co-active coaching: Changing business, transforming lives.* Boston, MA: Nicholas Brealey.

Krupnick, J. L., Sotsky, S. M., Simmens, S., Moyer, J., Elkin, I., Watkins, J., & Pilkonis, P. A. (1996). The role of the therapeutic alliance in psychotherapy and pharmacotherapy outcome: Findings in the National Institute of Mental Health Treatment of Depression Collaborative Research Program. *Journal of Consulting and Clinical Psychology, 64*(3), 532–539.

Luterman, D. (2008). *Counseling persons with communication disorders and their families* (5th ed.). Austin, TX: Pro-Ed.

Marziali, E., & Alexander, L. (1991). The power of the therapeutic relationship. *America Journal of Orthopsychiatry, 61*(3), 383–391.

Morse, J. M., & O'Brien, B. (1995). Preserving self: From victim, to patient, to disabled person. *Journal of Advanced Nursing, 21*(5), 886–896.

Page, J. L. (2015). The power of our stories: When we speak up and tell the stories of what we do, we give voice to our clients to tell their own. *The ASHA Leader, 20,* 6–7.

Pennebaker, J. W., & Seagal, J. D. (1999). Forming a story: The health benefits of narrative. *Journal of Clinical Psychology, 55*(10), 1243–1254.

Riley, J. (2002). Counseling: An approach for speech-language pathologists. *Contemporary Issues in Communication Science and Disorders, 29*, 6–16.

Safran, J. D., & Muran, J. (2000). *Negotiating the therapeutic alliance: A relational treatment guide.* New York, NY: Guilford Press

Silberman, S. (2015). *NeuroTribes: The legacy of autism and how to think smarter about people who think differently.* New York, NY: Avery.

Simmons-Mackie, N., & Damico, J. S. (2011). Counseling and aphasia treatment: Missed opportunities. *Topics in Language Disorders, 31*(4), 336–351.

Stein-Rubin, C., & Adler, B. T. (2012). Counseling and the diagnostic interview for the speech-language pathologist. In C. Stein-Rubin & R. Fabus (Eds.), *A guide to clinical assessment and professional report writing in speech-language pathology* (pp. 9–40). Clifton Park, NY: Delmar Cengage Learning.

Zebrowski, P. M., & Schum, R. L. (1993). Counseling parents of children who stutter. *American Journal of Speech-Language Pathology, 2*(2), 65–73.

2

Counselor Congruence

The good life is a process, not a destination.

—Carl Rogers, 1951

LEARNER OUTCOMES

After reading this chapter, the reader will be able to:

1. Discuss the two aspects of congruence.

2. Explain dissonance and role conflict.

3. Describe the various ways to develop congruence in one's life and for clients.

According to Carl Rogers (1951), one of the core conditions for a healthy therapeutic relationship is counselor *congruence*. Congruence is the consistency between the *ideal self* and the *actual self*. It is the alignment of our beliefs with our feelings and actions. Congruence requires *authenticity* and *genuineness* (the capacity to be real), which leads to a feeling of wholeness (Luterman, 2008).

In his book, *Counseling Clients With Communication Disorders and Their Families*, Luterman (2008) refers to the importance of counselor congruence:

> It is only when the counselor addresses and understands his or her own thoughts, emotions and reactions, and is secure enough not to need to be expert, that he or she is fully present for the client.

How we develop the *self* is of critical importance to our success as clinicians and at least as necessary as our academic knowledge. Developing ourselves will affect the way we talk to parents and provide support. Self-awareness influences the facilitator's *empathy*—the ability to be compassionate and caring. Empathy may be more effective than delivering a textbook explanation or speech. Clients will relate best to a clinician who is empathic, honest, and empowering, as well as supportive and knowledgeable.

Stein-Rubin, C., & Adler, B. T. *Counseling in Communication Disorders: Facilitating the Therapeutic Rehabilitation* (pp 9-23).
© 2017 Taylor & Francis Group.

OUR EARLY YEARS OF TRAINING

When we think back to our graduate school days, we recall that the emphasis in our training tended to be on academic content and how to become clinicians with the technical know-how. We focused on lectures, textbooks, projects, research, and papers. The focus was not on developing the *self* to be in touch with our own frailties, weaknesses, inadequacies, vulnerabilities, and limitations, all of which could have an impact on how we related to clients. As is typical of most graduate students, we were primarily aware of our fear and insecurity, which were related to areas where our training had been limited. This was particularly evident when we worked face-to-face with a client.

As relatively new clinicians and diagnosticians, we would frequently turn to a textbook for the explanations we thought we must deliver. We understood the importance of being well informed and well read, and at the time, our top priorities were carrying information in our heads and devoting our attention to our professional development. Although we were committed to helping and knew that our hearts were in the right place, we also knew we wanted to prove our knowledge and intelligence, that we had all the answers.

Yet across from us may have been a child and parent(s) who were looking to us for support and guidance. The reality of a session was sometimes startling. What would we, as beginning clinicians, do next? What would we say? How would we answer their questions? We learned quickly that without working on congruence, assessment and therapy would be overwhelming and fall short of what we hoped it would be.

MISSED MOMENTS

Students have told us that they often avoid asking clients and their families difficult questions. They fear their questions will be viewed as prying. We recall doing the same thing in our early years as new clinicians. Likewise, we relate to students when they tell us that they believe they may have missed an opportunity to explore a situation in greater depth. Their avoidance may have stemmed from their fear of the unknown. Specifically, the unknown relates to possible client reactions, questions, and comments. Furthermore, students talk about their uncertainty prioritizing information presented by the client and/or family members. They are fearful that they will deem something they hear as insignificant without inquiring further.

These missed moments have been called *counseling moments* (Roth & Worthington, 2011). They are the times in the dialogue when opportunities to have a more intimate and probing conversation reveal themselves. In retrospect, we now recognize these were times that our fears overpowered and paralyzed us. We were uncertain and insecure about dealing with the pain, worry, and fear on the faces of the parents, even as we wanted to help them.

We sometimes delivered too much information, and often information that was too technical. As a result, we ended up creating distance between the parents and ourselves. We did not understand why parents shut down. We may have even blamed them for not facing the situation and not accepting the realities of their child's needs and difficulties. It took us time to figure out what we'd done wrong in those situations. Steeped in fear, we had forgotten that everyone in the room was a human being and the importance of being in partnership. We may have been so focused on our own fears that we overlooked what it feels like to be overwhelmed and fearful, from their perspective. We neglected to address the parents' emotions.

IN THE PRESENT

Over the years, we have expanded and changed. Our healthiest and wisest selves have grown out of our desire to develop congruence and to seek self-awareness. The message of many masters has been driven home: To better understand who we are, we must continue to develop all parts of ourselves. We must accept our humanness, as well as the humanness of others, maintain authenticity and genuineness, and continue attempts to align our thoughts, feelings, and actions. We must nurture the ability to acknowledge what we see and the capacity to be real and say, "I hear your pain." We learned that our growth and our skills are not about having perfect knowledge and that our success would not emerge from an unbalanced scale. We had to learn to balance the art and the science of our profession.

As we have learned from the past and continue to learn from the present, we acknowledge that we are not the only experts. A collaborative model assumes the client is an equal partner in the process of exploring the difficulties presented. They are also equal partners in then finding alternative ways of navigating the problem (Fry & Cook, 2004; Fry & Farrants, 2003). The client is the expert on her own life, and there may be more than two experts in the room at a time, including family members. We have learned to acknowledge this partnership paradigm.

DISSONANCE IN ROLE CONFLICT

To fully understand congruence, we must examine the opposite, which is *dissonance*. Dissonance refers to the inconsistency between a person's beliefs or feelings and actions. For example, if an individual considers herself to be honest, yet lies and steals, there is inconsistency and therefore dissonance.

A form of dissonance is *role conflict*, coined by Joseph Sheehan (1970) in connection with stuttering, although it is applicable to any weakness or intrinsic challenge. For example, an individual may overuse reciting affirmations or personal mantras. That individual may look in the mirror and proclaim, "I'm perfect," which gives her an unrealistic and unreachable view causing her to feel dissonant. She may not really believe the mantra; it may feel false. On the other hand, if a person is trying to lose weight and she tells herself in the mirror, "I'm doing better than 3 months ago," that's a realistic positive affirmation that could bring her thoughts to a more adaptive place. Taking small reachable steps along the stepping stones of life gives us believable and reachable goals. Giving oneself a false sense of reality may lead to frustration and ultimately to giving up.

According to Sheehan (1970), until a person who stutters (PWS) identifies with herself as a PWS (as opposed to a fluent speaker), she won't be able to deal with her disorder in a healthy and adaptive way. That is, if a PWS believes that she is a "normal speaker" and interacts with others as though she's a "normal speaker," she will experience *role conflict* or dissonance between who she is as a speaker and how she falsely identifies her speech. Due to ensuing feelings of frustration, embarrassment, shame, and anger, her stuttering may increase. On the other hand, when we are fully transparent we can be more of who we are.

Sometimes we are not aware that dissonance is operating for ourselves or for our clients. We may not know why we have these uncomfortable feelings. These times might be opportunities for the clinician to acknowledge her own and/or the client's role conflict and bring greater awareness and congruence to the self and other.

Ask Yourself

1. Have you ever experienced an inconsistency between your beliefs and actions? Describe this situation and the impact it had on you.

2. Do you think of yourself in one way, yet others may describe you in a totally different way, which ends up surprising and confusing you? Explain this.

DEVELOPING CONGRUENCE

One question we might ask ourselves is, "How might we reach a state that would lead to greater congruence in our personal lives and in working with our clients?" If we indeed choose to achieve congruence, we must periodically stop, explore, look, review, and examine our daily lives. When we observe ourselves from the outside looking in, we may be surprised to find that there are answers, strategies, and a variety of ways to center ourselves and develop a more balanced state of being.

Some of us might ask, "How do we add more to our overcrowded and overwhelmed lives?" or "How will we find the time to learn about ourselves when we are spending all of our time learning the techniques and strategies for dealing with the struggles of others?" or "How does one establish balance?" Aren't the cries of "We don't have enough time!" and "Life is too stressful!" what we as human beings have in common? We hear students, faculty members, parents, children, and our family members and friends say, "There is no room in my schedule to do more!"

For our students, the struggle to balance their expectations of achieving their professional goals with the demands of personal responsibilities may be overwhelming. Although we all suffer from time constraints, the importance of gaining balance to become more centered, self-aware, and congruent is paramount for our work. Therefore, we decided to explore various areas in our lives where gaining balance facilitates greater congruence. The following tools may help us achieve greater congruence in our lives.

Balance and Technology

Using social media websites (e.g., Facebook, Twitter, and Instagram) is one of the most common activities among children and teenagers and has increased tremendously over the past few years (O'Keeffe & Clark-Peterson, 2011). Our students are also active participants in the world of social media and agree that technology is a double-edged sword. On one hand, it saves us time and allows us to reach out, connect with more people more often than we would otherwise, immediately answer questions that come up (instant gratification), and assist us in doing our research. On the other hand, technology has diminished our ability for human, face-to-face communication in real time. The constant interruptions of cell phones, e-mails, text messages, and social media may infringe on our inner peace and well-being and has been known to contribute to anxiety and stress. When we allow ourselves to become distracted by social media and text messaging we diminish our IQ for the task we are working on significantly (Ben-Shahar, 2010). We learn from the literature and from the news that technology, for many of us, has become an addiction.

Current research discusses the affliction of *social media anxiety*. Given the nature of social competition, cyberbullying, and resulting anxiety, parents must keep a tight rein on their children's involvement in these potentially harmful environments. All age groups participating in social media are exposed to what is happening in the lives of their peers. This fosters some unrealistic comparisons, and participants may become anxious and depressed about how everyone's photos and lives seem perfect and about the parties and other social events from which they were excluded (O'Keeffe & Clark-Peterson, 2011).

Although our students have commented about and agree with the benefits they experience using social media, they also acknowledge the downside. There are frequent misunderstandings resulting from not completing one's thoughts, not observing body language and eye contact, and not hearing vocal *prosody* (expression, rhythm, and inflection of the voice). Hurt feelings, anger, and anxiety ensue. Miscommunications inherent in technology may destroy relationships; for example, messages that go to the unintended recipient and result in, well…complications.

An added pressure for many of us is the 24-hour news cycle. Although we are frustrated and saddened by what we can now hear every minute of every day, we might find ourselves addicted to listening, and for many of us, our time is then consumed by one news program after another. This pattern becomes particularly detrimental when we watch news programs before going to bed. We may find that the stress of the news interferes with our sleep.

Ask Yourself

1. How many times have you or others used these phrases?
   - "Oh, that…I don't have the time for it any longer!"

   - "I forget what that's like."

   - "I haven't done that in such a long time; I miss it."

   - "I don't have time for my friends; I have too much work to do!"

2. As an experiment, choose a time of day to turn off your cell phone and computer. Take a break from technology to recharge your batteries. You will be surprised by how energized you feel after just an hour. When the hour is over, describe your feelings.

3. You may have heard about taking a news break, particularly before bed. American physician and holistic health advocate Dr. Andrew Weil (1995) suggests that you avoid watching the 11 p.m. news. He claims that once you make this change, you will sleep more peacefully and become more tranquil. Try it. See how you feel. Jot down the result(s).

4. Notice people who go on vacation and take their work and devices with them. How much true vacation time do they have? These same people may answer their phone when they're out to dinner. Instead of playing with their children, they may text and send e-mails. What is this behavior costing them? If you are one of these people, what are these behaviors costing you?

5. Notice the toll it takes on the family when a family member or friend works around the clock without a change of pace. How does this affect this person? How does it affect you?

Personal and Professional Boundaries

Learning to set *personal* and *professional boundaries* is central for one's health and well-being and requires mutual respect. Setting limits as to what one is willing to say and do in her daily life is essential. Many of us overextend ourselves because we are people-pleasers and do not know how to set limits to prevent ourselves from burning out. We might be afraid to say no to a request out of fear that we'll be thought of as selfish; we don't want to deal with the ensuing guilt.

The word *no* is important both internally and externally. Internally, it's about drawing boundaries to prevent harmful habits such as addiction or lack of safety. Externally, it's about maintaining our personal responsibility, integrity, and freedom; saying "no" is a brave and courageous act (Sills, 2013).

It's important to undertake the responsibilities we want and believe we are able to manage, rather than take on responsibilities that we feel pressured to accept. We may experience resentment when we find ourselves overextended, which may then interfere with our communication and relationships.

Sometimes, in clinical practice, we come to a point, after thoughtful consideration, when we must say no and set boundaries in our interaction with a client and family member. For example, clients or parents may push the professional boundaries in terms of telephone contact. They may call often or attempt to have long phone conferences during non-working hours. In those instances, it is important to design the alliance by clarifying professional protocols for the client or family member. We suggest letting them know that if they wish to talk to us between sessions, it is best to set up an appointment for a phone or in-person conference, so that we, as professionals, may be sure we are giving them our complete, uninterrupted, undivided attention.

Ask Yourself

1. Write about a situation in which you have had difficulty setting personal boundaries. Ask yourself, "What was I saying yes to?" and "What was I saying no to?" Also ask, "Am I overcommitting myself?"

2. Has this situation occurred in the professional arena as well? Explain.

Balance Through Mindfulness and Meditation

Mindfulness has been defined as "the practice of maintaining a nonjudgmental state of heightened or complete awareness of one's thoughts, emotions, or experiences on a moment-to-moment basis" (Merriam-Webster, n.d.). Mindfulness training keeps us focused on the "now" and encourages a reduction in multitasking. According to Ellen Langer (1989), when we are in a state of mindfulness, we may be more flexible in our thinking, open to new information, and aware of more than one perspective. Dr. Langer's research revealed that mindfulness is tied to good health and that the patients in nursing homes who were a part of her studies had an improvement in their overall health and an increase in longevity.

Meditation is a scientifically proven way to increase our mindfulness, or our attention to the present moment and to our thoughts. It has also proved to be a powerful means of promoting relaxation and well-being (Beauchemin, Hutchins, & Patterson, 2008).

When we *meditate*, we pay attention to the present moment and our breath and allow our thoughts to be waves that pass through our minds. In 1985, Herbert Benson, a cardiologist, encouraged meditation in hypertensive patients. Since then, meditation training has accompanied many medical treatments, including treatments for attention-deficit/hyperactivity disorder, cancer, depression, irritable bowel syndrome, anxiety, and depression.

In his book, *Full Catastrophe Living*, John Kabat-Zinn (2013) advocates for meditation training in hospitals, clinics, schools, and support groups. Kabat-Zinn runs extensive workshops to teach the benefits of meditation and suggests a variety of ways to incorporate the techniques into daily life. Now, thanks in large part to his efforts, it has become a mainstream practice in medicine. The medical literature has shown the benefits of what he termed *mindfulness-based stress reduction* in treating depression, chronic pain, cardiovascular disease, addictions, and a host of other ills.

As we embarked on our own personal and professional journeys, meditation became a significant part of our daily clinical and teaching practice. We usually begin our classes with several minutes of meditation. When we have asked our students how they felt after engaging in meditation, their responses included the following: "Relaxed"; "Centered"; "My headache is gone"; "I was overwhelmed when I arrived in class, and now I do not feel that way"; "Tranquil"; "Balanced"; and "At peace."

Beginning meditators often struggle with the practice of silence and stillness. In her book, *Eat, Pray, Love*, Elizabeth Gilbert (2006) describes her "monkey mind" during meditation, likening her uncontrolled thoughts to a monkey swinging from one tree to another. She envied her friend who sat in silence so easily for long periods of time. Fortunately, meditation becomes easier with practice.

The following are several suggestions for developing a basic meditation practice (there are many styles and techniques in addition to the ones noted here):

- *Sitting meditation*: Sit with your back supported, your feet flat on the floor, and your hands resting on your lap (palms up or middle fingers touching thumbs), or your left palm resting in your right palm. Focus on your breath. Eyes may be gently closed or slightly open, your gaze directed toward the floor. Count either your inhalations or your exhalations until 10, and then start again. Do not force your thoughts out. Allow the thoughts to pass through you as if they are waves moving across the mind and out. Work your way up to 10 to 20 minutes a day.

- *Meditation and music*: Sit following the instructions for sitting meditation and listen to soothing meditation music.

- *Walking meditation*: Find a comfortable place to walk in nature while focusing on your breath and/or listening to music suitable for meditation and calm. Keep your eyes looking forward.

- *Meditation while doing an activity*: Many athletes meditate while running or jogging. Any activity that allows you to be quiet and totally focused will work (Kabat-Zinn, 2013). You can even meditate while doing the dishes or making your bed.

- *Meditate while reclining*: Warning—don't fall asleep! However, once you're in a relaxed position on a mat, follow the sitting meditation instructions.

- *Meditation and mantras*: Some people choose a mantra, a word or phrase to repeat silently, over and over again, during meditation practice. Mantras may be of a spiritual nature or of your own creation as long as they help you to focus and be still.

Dr. Weil (1995) suggests a breathing routine for relaxation, waking, and falling asleep. He calls it *4–7–8*. The steps are as follows:

- Inhale through the nose to the count of 4 (keep the tongue tip on the alveolar ridge— the bumpy gum ridge at the roof of the mouth).

- Hold the breath to the count of 7.

- Exhale slowly through a small mouth opening to the count of 8.

- Do this 4 times. Stop. Repeat for another cycle of 4.

Everyone's count is different. Establish the count that works best for you.

Ask Yourself

After you have tried one or more of the preceding techniques several times, write about how meditation feels for you.

Balance Through Physical Exercise

Doing physical exercise is another critical step toward achieving balance. Many people tend to avoid exercising, but as noted by positive psychologists, without a regular physical fitness program, we are not functioning at even a baseline level. In other words, exercise does not get us operating above zero; rather, without it, our performance begins at a negative number (Ben-Shahar, 2010). Research has demonstrated that regular exercise (as little as 3 hours/week) can lower blood pressure and low-density lipoprotein ("bad") cholesterol; prevent and control weight gain and related illnesses such as diabetes and poor circulation; increase flexibility; reduce anxiety and depression, at least as effectively as psychiatric medications; facilitate alertness and attention; and even reduce the risk of cancer.

Ask Yourself

Notice how you feel after a workout and how much you can accomplish afterward. Describe.

Balance by Getting Enough Sleep

To become a high-functioning and congruent individual, it is essential to get enough sleep. In our society, people tend to believe that they can get by on little sleep. Maybe they can "get by," but they cannot thrive. According to the National Sleep Foundation (Hirshkowitz et al., 2015), by the age of 18 years old, 7 to 9 hours of sleep are needed each night in order not to be sleep deprived. According to positive psychologists, sleep deprivation significantly lowers a person's IQ (Ben-Shahar, 2010).

Balance by Taking Breaks

In their book *The Power of Full Engagement* (2003), Jim Loehr and Tony Schwartz explain that the human mind cannot maintain attention for much more than 90 minutes at a time. They suggest taking built-in breaks every hour and a half to maximize productivity: take a walk, listen to soothing or uplifting music, meditate, self-massage, do yoga, or stretch.

Ask Yourself

1. Notice how you nod out after studying or working for hours late at night without a restful break. What are the alternatives?

2. How does your mind feel after working diligently on a paper for 3 hours at a time?

The Wheel of Life

A wonderful life-balance tool is a diagram called the Wheel of Life. It's a circle divided into eight sections like a sliced pizza, each section representing a segment of our lives. Take a moment to look over the sample wheel (Figure 2-1).

Figure 2-1. The Wheel of Life.

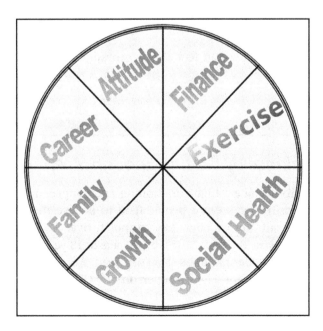

The categories in the picture are only an example. Create your own wheel with categories that feel relevant to your life. Divide each section into 10 horizontal sections by drawing horizontal lines. In each slice, color in a dark line across the number from 0 to 10 that corresponds to how satisfied you feel in that sphere of your life—10 is the best, and 0 is the worst. When you're finished, connect the dark lines, and you'll see a snapshot of your life; it might be quite ragged and could pose a very bumpy ride. When one aspect of your life is a 9 and another is a 3, chances are your life is out of balance. How congruent can one be if the ride is so bumpy (Whitworth, 2007)?

Ask Yourself

Choose a segment on the wheel (an aspect of your life) that you'd like to prioritize improving. Ask yourself the following questions:

1. What number would I like it to be?

2. What would that area of my life look like if it were that number?

3. Visualize and describe what that area of life would look like at the higher number.

4. How would this increase affect the rest of your wheel?

5. Name one small step you might take to bring this line to the number you want.

Connection

According to Seligman (2002), connection is one of the major pillars of well-being. Human beings are hardwired to need love and human interaction to thrive. As Albert Murphy (1981) said so eloquently:

> Every now and then something in our deeper selves enables us to realize what truly counts. In life, it is not a matter of what is in you or what is in me, but of what occurs between us. That divine spark of relationship may be the most fundamental life force of all.

Friendships can have a strong impact on our health, well-being, and our quality of life. From a health perspective, having friends influences our blood pressure, hormone stress levels, the quality of our sleep, and recuperation from physical injuries as we age. What affects us physically affects us emotionally. Good friends can offer hugs, a holding hand, and someone to talk to. According to research, having good friends can protect one from loneliness, emptiness, the risk of suicide, and alcoholism (Diener & Chan, 2011).

When it comes to friendships, quality surpasses quantity. In today's world, it is important for people to realize that thousands of friendships on Facebook do not replace time spent on cultivating and nurturing relationships. A study by the International Center for Media and Public Agenda (University of Maryland, 2011) examined the habits of young social media users. The study revealed that individuals who spend more time building online social networks experience a decrease in the quality of their real life friendships.

In the clinical arena, everyone involved in the therapeutic process will need support, from family, peers, the supervisors and therapists involved, and/or outside support groups. Our successes are the outgrowth of the combined efforts and partnerships established with other human beings. For most of us, we do not live or work in a vacuum; our congruence and centering is clearly enhanced by human connection.

If you want to go fast, go alone; if you want to go far, go together.

—African proverb

Ask Yourself

When was the last time you called an old and dear friend? How did you feel after the conversation?

Baby Steps

The goal in becoming more congruent is not perfection. It is about small shifts that may lead to big impacts. Think about undertaking one suggestion, mentioned in this chapter, for a few weeks, then moving on to incorporate another, and so on. It's worthwhile to reinforce reaching our goal by doing something that rewards our effort. When we allow ourselves the time to engage in whatever will be rewarding, we give ourselves a break, however brief, from our constant overwhelming routines. This positive reinforcement helps us gain a new and different perspective. When we take a step back, we have an opportunity to see things somewhat differently. We may balance our thinking and examine alternate possibilities to resolve our challenges. Then we're better able to be who we want to be for our families, partners, clients, and clients' families.

CONCLUSION

As *helpers* in a helping profession, we need to be open to personal centering. We need to sharpen our listening skills, expand our self-awareness, and have keener access to thoughts and feelings—our own and those of the people we know and work with. We need to accept the lessons life offers and realize that learning feeds the source that we become for others. We must develop strengths and understand our core values. We must know ourselves as we get to know our clients.

Ask Yourself

Complete the following and take the opportunity to apply the information from this chapter.

1. Are you someone who believes that personal growth is essential to doing your job well? Explain this based on what you have learned.

2. Explain in your own words how knowing more about yourself might have led you to handle:

   a. A *personal* situation differently.

   b. A *professional* situation differently.

3. Write down the kinds of things you have already done to further your self-awareness. If you haven't done much yet, which of these resonate for you?
   - Meditation training
   - Technology and news breaks
   - Getting enough sleep
   - Setting boundaries
   - Physical fitness and exercise
   - Yoga
   - Tai chi
   - Taking work breaks
   - Workshops, seminars, courses
   - Psychotherapy

- ○ Working with a life coach
- ○ Books (personal growth and development, self-awareness, psychology, and spirituality)

4. What energizes you? Think about what uplifts you, and how you may incorporate more of that in your daily life.

KEY CONCEPTS

- Congruence is the consistency between the ideal *self* and the actual *self* and depends on authenticity, genuineness, and the alignment of our beliefs with our feelings and actions.
- Congruence is also about achieving balance in all aspects of our lives (see Figure 2-1).
- Developing congruence is essential to being an effective facilitator.
- Dissonance is the opposite of congruence. It means there is an inconsistency between a person's beliefs and feelings and one's actions.
- Role conflict is a form of dissonance.
- Development of the *self* is of critical importance, at least as important as our academic knowledge.
- When a facilitator can address her own thoughts, emotions, and reactions, she can meet the needs of a client with greater understanding and presence.
- Clients will relate best to a clinician who is warm, supportive, and empowering, as well as knowledgeable.
- We need to allow time in our lives to focus on self-awareness and personal development as a means of achieving congruence. This is a lifelong process.
- There are numerous paths to personal development and self-awareness and to becoming a more congruent individual and professional.
- Small shifts lead to big impacts
  - ○ Reducing technology
  - ○ Drawing personal boundaries
  - ○ Mindfulness and meditation
  - ○ Physical exercise
  - ○ Getting enough sleep

○ Taking breaks
○ The Wheel of Life

REFERENCES

Beauchemin, J., Hutchins, T. L., & Patterson, F. (2008). Mindfulness meditation may lessen anxiety, promote social skills, and improve academic performance among adolescents with learning disabilities. *Complementary Health Practice Review, 13*(1), 34–45.

Ben-Shahar, T. (2010). *Foundations of positive psychology* [PowerPoint slides]. Retrieved from www.slideshare.net/ dadalaolang/1504-01intro?ref=http://positivepsychologyprogram.com/harvard-positive-psychology-course

Diener, E., & Chan, M. Y. (2011). Happy people live longer: Subjective well-being contributes to health and longevity. *Applied Psychology: Health and Well-Being, 3*(1), 1–43.

Fry, J., & Cook, F. (2004). Using cognitive therapy in group-work with young adults. In A. Packman, A. Meltzer, & H. F. M. Peters (Eds.), *Proceedings of the Fourth World Congress on Fluency Disorders, 2003. Theory, research and therapy in fluency disorders* (pp. 63–68). Nijmegen, The Netherlands: University of Nijmegen Press.

Fry, J., & Farrants, J. (2003). What's at stake? Adolescents' perceptions of the consequences of stuttering. In K.L. Baker & D. Rowley (Eds.), *Proceedings of the Sixth Oxford Dysfluency Conference* (pp. 275–278). York, United Kingdom: York Publishing Press.

Gilbert, E. (2006). *Eat, pray, love: One woman's search for everything across Italy, India, and Indonesia.* New York, NY: Viking.

Hirshkowitz, M., Whiton, K., Albert, S. M., Alessi, C., Bruni, O., DonCarlos, L....Adams Hilard, P. J. (2015). National sleep foundation's sleep time duration recommendations: Methodology and results summary. *Sleep Health, 1*(1), 40-43.

Kabat-Zinn, J. (2013). *Full catastrophe living, revised edition: How to cope with stress, pain and illness using mindfulness meditation.* London, United Kingdom: Hachette.

Langer, E. J. (1989). Minding matters: The consequences of mindlessness–mindfulness. *Advances in Experimental Social Psychology, 22,* 137–173.

Loehr, J. S., & Schwartz, T. (2003). *The power of full engagement: Managing energy, not time, is the key to high performance and personal renewal.* New York, NY: Free Press.

Luterman, D. (2008). *Counseling persons with communication disorders and their families* (5th ed.). Austin, TX: Pro-Ed.

Merriam-Webster (n.d.). Mindfulness. *Merriam-Webster.* Retrieved from www.merriam-webster.com/dictionary/ mindfulness.

Murphy, A. (1981). *Special children, special parents: Personal issues with handicapped children.* Englewood Cliffs, NJ: Prentice-Hall.

O'Keeffe, G. S., & Clark-Pearson, K. (2011). The impact of social media on children, adolescents, and families. *Pediatrics, 127*(4), 800–805. Retrieved from http://pediatrics.aappublications.org/content/127/4/800

Rogers, C. R. (1951). *Client-centered therapy: Its current practice, implications and theory.* Boston, MA: Houghton Mifflin.

Roth, F. P., & Worthington, C. K. (2011). *Treatment resource manual for speech-language pathologists.* Clifton Park, NY: Delmar Cengage Learning.

Seligman, M. E. (2002). *Authentic happiness: Using the new positive psychology to realize your potential for lasting fulfillment.* New York, NY: Free Press.

Sheehan, J. G. (1970). *Stuttering: Research and therapy.* New York, NY: Harper and Row.

Sills, J. (2013). The power of no. *Psychology Today.* Retrieved from www.psychologytoday.com/ articles/201310/the-power-no

University of Maryland, College Park. (2011). Students around the world report being addicted to media, study finds. *ScienceDaily.* Retrieved from www.sciencedaily.com/releases/2011/04/110405132459.htm.

Weil, A. (1995). *Spontaneous healing: How to discover and enhance your body's natural ability to heal itself.* New York, NY: Alfred A. Knopf.

Whitworth, L. (2007). *Co-active coaching: New skills for coaching people toward success in work and life.* Mountain View, CA: Davies-Black

3

Permission to Be Human

Forget your perfect offering/There is a crack, a crack in everything/That's how the light gets in.

—Leonard Cohen, 1992, track 1

LEARNER OUTCOMES

After reading this chapter, the reader will be able to:

1. Explain the importance and relevance, as a clinician, of accepting negative emotions as part of the human condition.

2. Become familiar with the ways to deliver painful news.

3. Identify ways to counsel parents about giving children permission to access and relate their negative emotions.

4. Name the different stages of the Grief Cycle and explain how this relates to counseling clients and families.

5. Discuss the various causes of fear of success with respect to their clients.

My (CSR) grandchildren and young clients often express anger and frustration. On that note, I'd like to share a story with you about my 2-year-old granddaughter, Leah, who has been struggling with the arrival of her new baby sister. As everyone around her makes a fuss about the baby, Leah often becomes furious and tends to act out. On these occasions, I remind her of a book that I gave her, *When Sophie Gets Angry—Really, Really Angry* (Bang, 1999), and I ask her if she feels angry like Sophie. My granddaughter always pauses, her facial expression softens, and she responds by recalling the story, for example, "Sophie's really, really angry; Leah's also angry." We then go into the kinds of things my granddaughter might do when she's very angry, such as running really fast or punching the sofa.

Stein-Rubin, C., & Adler, B. T. *Counseling in Communication Disorders: Facilitating the Therapeutic Rehabilitation* (pp 25-47).
© 2017 Taylor & Francis Group.

Student-clinicians and beginning clinicians may be unaware of the importance of giving their clients the *permission to be human.*[1] The student-clinicians may have responded to Leah, as family members might, with comments instructing her how to behave. Generally, this would serve to make her feel angrier and cause her to act out more. Parents and clinicians are often overwhelmed when their children or clients become angry. Once we take the perspective that anger is a normal human emotion and learn to acknowledge it (not only in children but in adults as well), these reactions become less frightening.

Experiencing painful emotions is part of the human condition. In this chapter, we attempt to illuminate the importance of being honest with others and with ourselves about our negative emotions and how this transparency actually helps human beings like themselves better. When we view ourselves and others as whole, despite negative emotions, we have reached a pivotal milestone in reaching our full potential. We, as clinicians, supervisors, and instructors, need to be aware of this concept and to practice nonjudgmental acceptance of the full range of human emotions. Acknowledging these in our clients and their families builds trust and self-esteem and deepens the therapeutic relationship.

This story illustrates what positive psychologist Tal Ben-Shahar (2010) means when he talks about giving others and ourselves the permission to be human. Acknowledging permission to be human is integral to setting us on the path toward well-being, happiness, and self-esteem. Giving others and ourselves that permission also means that, within all of us, there needs to be a space for positive emotions as well as for difficult ones. Empathy, by definition, is "the feeling that you understand and share another person's experiences and emotions: the ability to share someone else's feelings" (Merriam-Webster, n.d.). Carl Rogers (1951) considered empathy as one of the three essential ingredients for a positive therapeutic relationship (see Chapter 2).

Ask Yourself

1. In order to develop greater sensitivity to the feelings of someone experiencing and living with a disability, select a handicapping condition such as restriction of the use of one arm, stuttering, limp, word retrieval struggle, and/or a hearing loss. Live life with this limitation during the weekend. Describe the feelings and observations.

2. In order to build trust and learn how to ask for support, engage in the blindfold exercise in twos. One person covers his eyes and tells the other how to guide him or her down the hallway safely.

---

[1] The phrases *permission to be human* and *empathy* are similar in meaning and will be used interchangeably throughout this chapter.

Leaning Into the Discomfort

When an individual takes the time to process negative emotions, rather than running away from them, in the field of social work, this is called *leaning into the discomfort*. Leaning into the discomfort, or giving ourselves the permission to be human, is counterintuitive in our society where uncomfortable emotions are eschewed and people are encouraged to smile and be happy. The literature, however, indicates otherwise (Hutz, 2010).

It is commonly known that one of the most stressful experiences for all human beings is public speaking. Even the most famous speakers, as well as entertainers such as Barbra Streisand and Adele, experience stage fright before a performance. When we, as instructors, go into class to teach courses or to conduct presentations, we frequently feel anxious or nervous about delivering the lecture. Earlier in our careers, we handled the problem by saying, "I am not going to be nervous; there is no room for anxiety here."

The Pink Elephant

The famous psychological study of the *pink elephant* (Wegner, Schneider, Carter, & White, 1987) illustrates this phenomenon. If we are told *not* to think of a pink elephant over and over again, we are destined to have pink elephants invade our imagination. Over time, we have learned to lean into the discomfort, even though it made us squirm. We honored the uncomfortable emotions, became curious about them, and let them be there without judging. Curiosity about uncomfortable emotions may lead to positive change. Although overwhelming anxiety before a presentation may be debilitating, a bit of anxiety may actually keep us alert, excited, and alive in the present moment. Once we give ourselves permission to experience the fear, admit it, and not try to hide from it or deny it, we often emerge from the other side feeling freer. This process is honest, active, and courageous (Box 3-1).

Box 3-1

We will never forget Lazaro Arbos, the young man who stuttered and tried out for the TV show *American Idol*. He openly declared himself a stutterer and explained the nature of his disorder to the judges and the world. He told his story; spoke of his childhood pain, isolation, and loneliness; and miraculously made the cut! Lazaro proceeded to compete until he was one of the top five final contenders. He sang like a bird and, as is typical, did not stutter when he sang. Lazaro gave himself permission to be human, in front of the viewers worldwide, and won the hearts of the judges and audience with his raw authenticity. We will refer again to Lazaro Arbos in Chapter 8.

Many persons who stutter (PWS) in time come to agree that stuttering is an opportunity—a gift. The struggle they have in communication has afforded them compassion, patience, kindness, and courage. Many PWS move on to become speech-language pathologists, who then work with individuals who stutter. They supervise student-clinicians and teach courses on the topic. Although their speech may be extremely disfluent, they are often selected for these professional roles over fluent speakers. These individuals take the opportunity to honor and teach their students and clients how to openly acknowledge familiar painful emotions and struggles surrounding their stuttering.

ACCEPTING THE FULL RANGE OF EMOTIONS

Ben-Shahar (2010) says that all emotions flow through the same emotional pipeline. Without giving ourselves permission to feel our uncomfortable, difficult, or negative emotions, we block the pathway for positive ones like love, gratitude, joy, and awe. Accepting our full range of emotions is how we achieve self-acceptance and self-love, crucial goals for our work. Until this is achieved, we will not be able to get down to the business of problem solving with our clients or ourselves.

Experiencing our emotions has healing properties. Yet most of us feel like there must be something wrong or defective within us when negative emotions occur. Our clients most likely feel similarly for their own reasons; nevertheless, when we avoid and suppress uncomfortable emotions, it gives these feelings more power (Ben-Shahar, 2010). In reality, our emotions or feelings are just feelings; they are neither good nor bad, they just *are* (Burns, 1999). We cannot change a feeling by snapping our fingers, whether the feeling is our own or someone else's. We can simply hear it, be with it, and try our best to understand it. At the same time, feeling our painful emotions does not imply we passively resign to them; it is about accepting them (Box 3-2).

Box 3-2

I (CSR) recall a story about my teenage son. His new kitten was dying, and he expressed great fear. I remember feeling somewhat confused about why he expressed fright rather than sadness. When I asked him why he felt scared, he replied, "I'm scared of how sad I'm going to feel when Nala dies." My son's profound admission went straight to my heart and taught me a great deal about accessing, processing, and verbalizing emotions. My son, in his reaction, also highlighted for me how much we, as adults, avoid talking about the unpleasant stuff. This experience became an inspiration for me as I trained and taught my students.

As we work with and learn to love and respect (at least to be okay with) all the parts of ourselves, we can extend that compassion and understanding outward to others. This is the love that the clinician shows the client, the unconditional acceptance of him with his full range of emotions—the good, the bad, and the ugly (Box 3-3).

Box 3-3

Some years ago a colleague who is a psychologist asked me (BTA) to work with a 5-year-old girl who had been diagnosed as a selective mute. The child refused to speak in school and refused to engage with this therapist. Our plan was to see whether she would connect with me at all, and once on her way, if successful, we would all work together.

When this little girl entered the room, she avoided eye contact and refused to speak. We sat on the floor and played silently with the toys she selected. I spoke in a soft voice and avoided questions. At one point, she stood up, picked a toy and sat down with her back to me. My comment was, "Oh, I guess we can each play separately with our backs to each other." During the next session, we maintained the same positions. After a little while I whispered to her the name of my doll and told her that it was okay to whisper in this room if she wanted to. Suddenly, she whispered her doll's name. From that day on, we sat back-to-back and inch by inch eventually ended up face-to-face. Our voices grew stronger, and we talked more. At the same time, no one ever made a fuss about it; we kept it all very calm.

Eventually when the child returned to work with the psychologist, she interacted appropriately, and we agreed that the team effort was invaluable. Our client entered the first grade as a communicator and did not require our services any longer.

Mister Rogers, the famous children's TV host, encouraged children to feel their negative emotions and acknowledge them. He taught us, as parents and clinicians, how to help our children achieve and enhance this skill (Box 3-4).

Box 3-4

WHAT DO YOU DO WITH THE MAD THAT YOU FEEL?

by Fred M. Rogers

What do you do with the mad that you feel

When you feel so mad you could bite?

When the whole wide world seems oh, so wrong...

And nothing you do seems very right?

What do you do? Do you punch a bag?

Do you pound some clay or some dough?

Do you round up friends for a game of tag?

Or see how fast you go?

It's great to be able to stop

When you've planned a thing that's wrong,

And be able to do something else instead

And think this song:

I can stop when I want to

Can stop when I wish.

(continued)

BOX 3-4 (CONTINUED)
I can stop, stop, stop any time. And what a good feeling to feel like this, And know that the feeling is really mine. Know that there's something deep inside That helps us become what we can. For a girl can be someday a woman And a boy can be someday a man. What Do You Do with the Mad that You Feel?
© McFeely-Rogers Foundation. Used with permission.

Fred Rogers served as an acclaimed role model to help children learn about experiencing the full range of their emotions, to love and regard themselves as special despite negative emotions, and to learn how to manage these negative feelings. Children are all too often admonished for showing negative emotions and are then taught to stifle them. We find it is worthwhile to encourage children to watch the recordings of his show and to read his books. Unfortunately, Rogers passed away several years ago; however, his legacy lives on.

The Impact of Other's Reactions

Notice the many ways people you know respond when you share your negative experiences and emotions. Do the other individuals trivialize or avoid your uncomfortable feelings? Although this response may be well intended, it is possible that these comments inadvertently imply that you are overreacting. This reply may lead you to feel invalidated, and that your problem is not important enough. Furthermore, other reactions could suggest you are not doing enough, working hard enough, trying persistently enough—that in some way *you* are not enough (Kimsey-House, Kimsey-House, Sandahl, & Whitworth, 2011).

Ask Yourself

1. Identify one or more emotions you might be afraid to feel. How can you cope with the fear?

2. How do you handle your uncomfortable emotions?

EMPATHY VERSUS SYMPATHY

At this point, it is important to distinguish between empathy and sympathy. Our students often struggle with understanding the difference between the two concepts. Empathy empowers and sympathy disempowers. To have *empathy* for another human is to feel with them and understand what the other person is experiencing, describing, and sharing. On the other hand, when we have *sympathy* for someone else, we feel sorry for the person and her struggles. Although we can feel sorry and sad for someone going through a difficult time, we don't want to treat him in a pitying way that would be demeaning and diminish courage. Brown (2006) points out that empathy rarely starts with the words, "At least…" where the listener gives the other person the bright side or tries to problem solve. A more effective response might be, "I appreciate that you shared this with me."

When a client relates his situation to a clinician, the clinician's well-intentioned response is all too frequently, "I understand." Clients and family members have been known to respond to this comment, "No, you don't understand. No one can understand unless they have gone through this." An alternative phrase for "I understand" might be, "I hear what you're saying, and it sounds like this is difficult." When we feel heard, understood, and cared about, it gives individuals a feeling of love, belonging, acceptance, and support (Thieda, 2014).

We do not have to have the same experiences as those for whom we provide therapy. We do not have to live with a particular child with special needs, day in and day out, to understand the parents' struggle. Yet we do need to listen and to relate within ourselves, to some type of similar experience, so that we may show up as empathic, warm, supportive, and caring.

Ask Yourself

Describe a time when you would have appreciated someone empathizing with you about your difficulty rather than feeling sorry for you.

JOINING WITH

One of our most important roles is *joining with* our clients and families in their experience. By joining with the client, we create an inviting and spacious place for him to be in the full experience of his life (Kimsey-House et al., 2011). It is essential for the clinician to recognize these emotions and resist the urge to fix them, make them go away, or dodge them (Oriah Mountain Dreamer, 1999). It is most challenging for a clinician to learn to be *present* or fully attuned to the immediate moment with a client or family's tears and pain.

As caring individuals in a helping profession, our instinct is to cheer up our clients, make their sadness go away, and find a "bright side" for them. Although well-intentioned, this *Pollyanna attitude* implies that pain is taboo (Ben-Shahar, 2010). Avoiding difficult and negative emotions will surely alter the space. It is this space that serves as a container to hold the relationship (Whitworth, 2007). Therefore, to be with, or join with the client, is an active process where you are fully engaged in the present moment.

Janice Fialka (1997), a parent of a child with special needs, expressed her need for the speech-language pathologist to join with her in the moment without judgment, advice, or offering technical information. By doing this, Fialka requests permission, for her son and for herself, to be human and that becomes a critical part of the healing process. We all need a safe space in our lives, at least one safe person, where we grant ourselves this permission (Box 3-5).

Box 3-5

ADVICE TO PROFESSIONALS WHO MUST "CONFERENCE CASES"

by Janice Fialka
www.danceofpartnership.com
Before the case conference,
I looked at my almost five-year-old son
and saw a golden-haired boy
who giggled at his baby sister's attempts to clap her hands,
who charmed adults by his spontaneous hugs and hellos,
who often became a legend in places visited
because of his exquisite ability to befriend a few special souls,
Who often wanted to play "peace marches"
And who, at the age of four,
went to the Detroit Public Library
requesting a book on Martin Luther King.
After the case conference,
I looked at my almost five-year-old son.
He seemed to have lost his golden hair.
I saw only words plastered on his face,
Words that drowned us in fear,
Words like:
Primary Expressive Speech and Language Disorder,
Severe Visual Motor Delay,
Sensory Integration Dysfunction,
Fine and Gross Motor Delay,
Developmental Dyspraxia and RITALIN now.
I want my son back. That's all.
I want him back now. Then I'll get on with my life.
If you could see the depth of this pain
If you feel this sadness

(continued)

BOX 3-5 (CONTINUED)

Then you would be moved to return
Our almost five-year-old son
who sparkles in sunlight despite his faulty neurons.
Please give us back my son
undamaged and untouched by your labels, test results,
descriptions and categories.
If you can't, if you truly cannot give us back our son
Then just be with us
quietly, gently, softly.
Sit with us and create a stillness
known only in small, empty chapels at sundown.
Be there with us
as our witness and as our friend.
Please do not give us advice, suggestions, comparisons or
another appointment. (That is for later.)
We want only a quiet shoulder upon which to rest our heads.
If you cannot give us back our sweet dream
then comfort us through this evening.
Hold us. Rock us until morning light creeps in.
Then we will rise and begin the work of a new day.

© 1997 Janice Fialka

Robert Ball (2014) was a judge in a contest in which young children submitted stories about caring. The story in Box 3-6 won and is another example of acceptance and joining with, describing how a 4-year-old boy joins with an elderly gentleman as he mourns the loss of his wife.

BOX 3-6

A 4-year-old child's neighbor was an elderly gentleman who had recently lost his wife. Upon seeing him cry, the little boy went into the gentleman's yard, climbed onto his lap, and just sat there. When his mother asked what he had said to the neighbor, he said, "Nothing. I just helped him cry" (Ball, 2014).

Many religions designate a time to be with a person who is in mourning. One example of this type of empathy and joining with is found in the Jewish tradition of sitting Shiva. In Judaism, when one suffers a loss in the immediate family, the family members sit at home for 7 days while visitors come to pay their respects. The visitors are not obligated to speak

Figure 3-1. Sheehan's iceberg metaphor for the associated emotions for individuals who stutter.

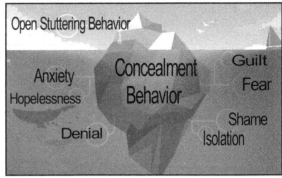

or to do anything. It is just about being with the mourner. Often individuals sit in silence when the mourner begins to speak about loss, his loved one, and related memories. The Shiva, meaning *seven* (days), is cathartic for the mourners as they experience a week with their friends, family, and acquaintances joining with them.

REPRESSED EMOTIONS INTENSIFY IN STUTTERING

A famous and powerful analogy for how repressed human emotions intensify and interfere when not addressed is Joseph Sheehan's (1970) iceberg metaphor as it relates to stuttering. According to Sheehan, "Stuttering is like an iceberg, with only a small part above the waterline and a much bigger part below…Successful suppression is what maintains and perpetuates the stuttering."

Up until Sheehan's model, most speech-language pathologists treated only the actual stuttering characteristics, the part above the waterline. They largely ignored the submerged emotions. We were trained to avoid the emotional component of stuttering with the rationale that if you could "control" the stuttering, the individual would become more fluent and the emotional component would dissipate.

Unfortunately, by treating only the stuttering symptoms, even if the individual achieved greater fluency, there was a high level of relapse. By ignoring the coexisting painful emotions found in confirmed individuals who stutter, the ignored emotions intensified further complicating the disorder.

Fortunately over time, we have learned to treat the emotional well-being of our clients. The literature also indicates the importance of conversing with preschool children who stutter about their related emotions and attitudes, as well as coaching parents on how to talk to their children about talking. Logan and Yaruss (1999) stress the importance of focusing on the quality of life while addressing overt stuttering symptoms. Likewise, we have also come to realize that, to do this, the facilitator must also work on his own iceberg (Figure 3-1).

Ask Yourself

Think of an event that occurred in your life for which you may have repressed your feelings. What did you do?

CHALLENGING CONVERSATIONS

A study examining the interactions between clinicians and their adult patients suffering from aphasia revealed that the clinicians usually avoided counseling opportunities and emotional conversations. Instead they discussed facts, engaged in superficial chitchat, used humor to deflect emotional reactions, and changed the focus to treatment tasks (Simmons-Mackie & Damico, 2011).

Engaging in difficult conversations is often challenging and evokes anxiety in many of us. Nevertheless, it is necessary to provide a safe space to explore the many emotions of our clients and their families. These conversations help sustain treatment goals.

We need to reflect on why we are uncomfortable. If our discomfort stems from feeling we are out of our element, we may need to enlist the help of other professionals. If our awkward feelings come more from being with others' painful experiences, we need to confront that, lean into our own discomfort, and experience it. Additional experience, with an open mind in these situations, will help desensitize us to discomfort.

It has been our clinical experience that many clients and family members find their ways into our offices rather than, or before, seeking other professional assistance (e.g., mental health counselor, neurologist, otolaryngologist). It seems that for many people, seeing a speech-language pathologist is less threatening and stigmatizing than an evaluation by another one of the other health-related professionals. Furthermore, our clinical setting is often the first place that an individual divulges personal information and problems.

Since this scenario is fairly typical in clinical interactions, it is important that the speech-language pathologist prepare cognitively and emotionally for its occurrence. As clinicians, we must be mindful and self-manage our own emotions, so that we are confident to move forward and engage in these conversations. It is only when we have developed the self-awareness and courage to pursue emotional exploration with our clients and families that we may be in the best service to the people with whom we work. For additional information on this topic, we refer the reader to the book *Difficult Conversations* by Douglas Stone, Bruce Patton, and Sheila Heen (2010).

In the beginning, our clients may arrive at our door fearful about what to expect and about what they may be told. Our responsibility goes beyond establishing rapport. It is about creating a sense of trust, safety, comfort, honesty, and engendering hope, from the start, as early on as the first diagnostic interview. There are several ways to cultivate a deep therapeutic relationship. These methods include the following attitudes and techniques:

- Our timing is critical with respect to delivering painful news and is largely dependent on the nature and depth of the therapeutic relationship.

- Give clients and family members the permission to be human and the opportunity to fully express their painful emotions without fear of judgment.
- Use deep nonjudgmental listening.
- Use sensitive language.
- Acknowledgment of strengths
- Maintain an open curious attitude.
- Be mindful of nonverbal communication (body language, facial expression, and positioning).
- Use shoulder-to-shoulder seating rather than including a barrier between you and the client (Axline, 2014; Kimsey-House et al., 2011; Robinson, 2015; Rogers, 1951).

Robinson (2015) went on to encourage us to cultivate relationships with our clients and their families before delivering difficult news. "It's always easier to hear the negative from a close person than from a stranger," says Robinson, "so it's preferred to cultivate a relationship with the client and family before delivering serious news." Once the family member is given some time to process the information, he may come to his own conclusion. The clinician may then add to the parent's own observations and realizations. By giving the family member the opportunity to develop his own ideas, we increase the likelihood that he will own the solution and follow through, rather than if he was simply told (Kimsey-House et al., 2011; Rogers, 1951). The importance of honesty cannot be overemphasized when communicating with clients and families from the outset—clients prefer this (Axline, 2014).

Ask Yourself

1. Were you ever the person who had to deliver uncomfortable news? Describe your feelings. How was the timing?

2. Have you ever observed someone delivering or receiving serious news? Write down your observations about the interaction and the timing.

3. Describe any other personal experiences you have had with either delivering or receiving painful news? What was the impact?

Counseling Parents About "Talking About Talking"

As facilitators, we need to train parents in the importance of engaging in difficult conversations with their children. For example, clinicians who work with children must teach parents about "talking about talking" (Ainsworth & Fraser, 1988). Parents of children who stutter are most concerned that their discussion of their children's difficulty with fluency will exacerbate their children's stuttering (Johnson & Associates, 1959). Even though this belief is common it is not supported by the current literature (Logan & Yaruss, 1999; Yaruss, 2010).

According to Logan and Yaruss (1999), the most productive thing parents can do to alleviate their child's stuttering is to engage in conversations that are open, nonjudgmental, and genuinely curious. These conversations give parents further insight into their child's experience (Logan & Yaruss, 1999). In addition, parents also may make assumptions about what their child is thinking and feeling and are then surprised to find out that their own beliefs were not the reality at all.

Parents may learn how to authentically reassure their children based on these open conversations. For example, a parent may discover that her child fears something that is unfounded and may have no idea what it is until a conversation is started. A child may believe he is "stupid," "bad," or has "something wrong with my brain." The parent would be unable to manage this faulty thinking, and reassure the child without insight into his child's thoughts. The parent may also need the reassurance and assistance from the clinician to learn how to communicate with the child about these fears (Logan & Yaruss, 1999).

Counseling Parents About Negative Emotions

As discussed earlier, it is crucial for clinicians to help their clients and family members to be transparent about their negative emotions. It is also critical for clinicians to counsel parents on how to help their children access and discuss their own painful feelings. Logan and Yaruss (1999) outlined the following three factors for parents to be aware of when talking with their children about stuttering. These factors are applicable to other speech-language and hearing disorders as well as to everyday situations:

1. *Affective factors*—It is important that parents understand the way their emotions and reactions to their child's stuttering influence their child's coping strategies. Emotions such as guilt, embarrassment, shame, and panic need to be highlighted for parents so that these feelings and attitudes do not interfere with the parent's reactions to their child.

2. *Behavioral factors*—Parents need to pay attention to their nonverbal behavior such as eye contact, facial expression, and body language (Gottwald & Starkweather, 1995). The clinician may help nonverbal behaviors through the use of videotaping and can then be reviewed in a clinical conference with parents.

3. *Cognitive factors*—It is important to note that parents may have a discrepancy between their thoughts and feelings about their child's stuttering. For example, although parents may cognitively know that they did not cause their child's stuttering, they may still feel somehow responsible and guilty. It's the clinician's responsibility to call out these incongruities to the parents and discuss their ambivalence.

The importance of educating parents in the facts about stuttering or about any other communication disorder cannot be overestimated. Once parents gather information about their child's struggle, some of their inaccurate beliefs, anxieties, and other emotions may be dispelled (Logan & Yaruss, 1999).

It is also essential to consider parental feelings in connection to their child's stuttering. The clinician may want to delineate for the parent some typical feelings of other parents who share their situation. This helps parents realize that their feelings are normal and helps relieve any possible secondary guilt about what they are experiencing. Another way to diminish parental guilt is to encourage parents to focus on what's working in the present and on what they are doing to alleviate their child's difficulties. There is an abundance of literature, through the Stuttering Foundation and the National Stuttering Project, to supplement the counseling that we do with parents (Zebrowski & Schum, 1993).

Heightening Client Awareness

One of our goals as speech-language and hearing clinicians is to heighten client awareness of their thoughts and emotions; we need to stay present to the conversation and expand upon it. When a client exhibits signs of emotion such as anger or sadness, a clinician may ask what the client's thoughts are and to describe what he is feeling. If a clinician notices that a client is anxious or particularly upset about his communication, the clinician might ask the client to sit with the feeling and give him the opportunity to feel it. The clinician may then want to move on to asking the client to notice the times when he experiences these emotions related to his communication. As the intensity dissipates, there is usually a shift in the client from a position of automatic reaction to a place of awareness and feeling lighter (Riley, 2002).

WE ARE ALL CONNECTED

It is natural for people to view themselves as different from others, and in many ways we are all different from each other. Yet in truth, we have also witnessed that our humanness makes us more alike than different. Across cultures, socioeconomic levels, gender differences, and generations, we are all more the same than one would expect.

Even though each culture has different traditions and customs, food preferences and rules, behaviors and rituals, there are nevertheless similarities among all people. No matter where we come from, there is a strong commonality to the range of our emotions, our hopes, our aspirations, and our dreams.

The Grief Cycle

All human beings are also connected through a loss or a death in the family. Elizabeth Kübler-Ross (1969), in her book *On Death and Dying,* discusses five stages of grief that all human beings go through in response to loss and catastrophic events. The cycle is also applicable when a person or family member experiences a communication or hearing disorder. For the family whose child has special needs, there is the death of a dream—the dream of having a typically developing child or the dream of what a child who lost his skills might have become.

If we study these stages as clinicians, we become more cognizant, sensitive, and empathetic to understanding what a client or family goes through when diagnosed with a speech-language disorder and beyond. Equally important, studying these stages helps us understand where we might be at should we go through a grieving process.

It is important to note that no two individuals are the same, and everyone grieves differently. An individual may not go through these stages in precisely this order. Furthermore, one may cycle back to previous stages and then move forward once again. It is essential that we give our clients and ourselves the permission to be human for stages or cycles of emotions as well as for isolated painful emotions.

The following are the five stages described by Elizabeth Kübler-Ross (1969):

1. *Denial*—The first reaction to a catastrophic event is to hide from the situation and pretend it does not exist. We often see parents who are concerned about their child's development. They may bring their child to us as a result of a referral. Unfortunately, the parent may refuse to accept our diagnosis or description of a child's problem. They may not understand why a teacher recommended additional supports or a change in the classroom. The parent may not be willing or ready to believe and accept that there is a problem that needs to be addressed.

2. *Anger*—As the wall of denial begins to wear away, the pain resurfaces as anger. This anger may be directed toward us, as clinicians (in addition to family, friends, strangers, etc.). When we as clinicians understand where the anger stems from in terms of the grief cycle, we may refrain from taking it personally and meet the client where he is. In addition, the client may feel guilty for his feelings of anger, which may be directed at the deceased, for dying and leaving them, or at the family member with the disorder. This compounds the feelings of anger, with secondary guilt causing more of a struggle for the client.

3. *Bargaining*—In an effort to regain control, we may immerse ourselves in *should statements* (e.g., "I should have checked into this earlier and prevented it," "I should have been a better son [mother, father, etc.]," or "I should have done more."). This stage may also involve bargaining with a higher power, offering to abstain from something or to do something major, in exchange for sparing the person or family member.

4. *Depression*—This is the phase where we actually mourn the loss of the person, or the person the way we once knew him. Kindness, understanding, patience, and a hug are prescriptions for this phase of the process.

5. *Acceptance*—Not everyone in a catastrophic situation reaches this stage. One may be stuck in denial, another in anger. It is important to note that *acceptance* does not mean happiness. It is actually a period marked by withdrawal and must be distinguished from depression.

Ask Yourself

1. Do you agree with the statement, "People are more alike than different"? Provide an example.

2. Describe a time in your life or in someone else's in terms of the grief cycle.

FAMILY CAREGIVERS

In the work we do with adult clients who have experienced a life-altering event such as a stroke, we frequently find ourselves working with their caregivers. Several qualitative and quantitative research studies indicate that caregivers play an integral role in client success (Christensen, Skaggs, & Kleist, 1997; Michallet, Le Dorze, & Tétreault, 2001; Visser-Meily et al., 2006). They are communication partners, overseers of the client's day-to-day living, coordinators of the client's affairs, and "therapists" for stimulating and generalizing progress. As part of the client's family, the dynamics and stresses of that relationship affect the caregiver's well-being (Logan & Yaruss, 1999). We need to be empathetic about the toll this may take on the caregiver's life.

Results of a survey of 38 family caregivers, regarding patients with aphasia, suggest that once the caregiver receives bad news, his needs and attitudes change over time. It is important for us to be cognizant of the cycle of stages regarding these changes, which can help clinicians to support clients, families, and their caregivers. For more detailed information on this topic, we refer the reader to the article "Counseling the Caregiver" (Hunting Pompon, Burns, & Kendall, 2015).

UNFOUNDED REACTIONS

There are times when any one of us may overreact to an individual and/or a situation, particularly if we are already dealing with repressed or uncomfortable emotions. Parents may end up overreacting with the clinician and expressing themselves unpleasantly. Their reactions may be due to frustration, anger, sadness, and guilt related to their child's struggles. The parents' behavior may not necessarily be related to us or to our work yet we may take their words too personally and develop our own feelings of hurt, defensiveness, and frustration about their attitude (Box 3-7).

BOX 3-7

A speech-language clinician was having a particularly difficult day for personal reasons. On that same day, a parent was frustrated with his child's therapy. The parent expressed his upset to the clinician. The parent expressed that his child was not progressing rapidly enough. The clinician, who was already feeling vulnerable, overreacted to the parent's words and took them far more personally than was warranted.

Often, parents overlook and forget that their patience is required in the therapeutic process. At the same time, this is one of the reasons it is so important for clinicians to do their own work on recognizing their emotions and what the source is for those feelings. As we work on our listening and language in the following chapters, we discuss how to diffuse these upsets.

Ask Yourself

1. Recall a time when you blamed someone else for your own repressed emotion. What was the outcome?

2. Recall a time when someone blamed you for something you did not do. How did that feel?

3. Who is your "safe person?" Is it your mother, sister, friend, significant other? Or is it yourself?

FEAR OF SUCCESS

We have noticed within ourselves, our clients and their family members, our own families, friends, colleagues, and students that we all may experience a degree of *fear of success*. When individuals see things going in a positive direction, they become anxious and may not know why. We have learned that it is just as important for us to give ourselves permission to feel positive emotions as it is to experience negative emotions.

> What is required for many of us, paradoxical though it may sound, is the courage to tolerate happiness (in the present) without self-sabotage…The greatest crime we commit against ourselves is not that we may deny and disown our shortcomings, but that we deny and disown our greatness—because it frightens us. (Branden, 1995)

Branden's quote creates a paradox. What would make us fear our success and happiness as much as our fear of failure and unhappiness? Why would happiness require courage?

Marianne Williamson (1996) expresses fear of success in Box 3-8.

Box 3-8

Our deepest fear is not that we are inadequate. Our deepest fear is that we are powerful beyond measure. It is our light, not our darkness that most frightens us. We ask ourselves, "Who am I to be brilliant, gorgeous, talented, fabulous?" Actually, who are you not to be? You are a child of God. Your playing small does not serve the world. There is nothing enlightened about shrinking so that other people won't feel insecure around you. We are all meant to shine, as children do. We were born to make manifest the glory of God that is within us. It's not just in some of us; it's in everyone. And as we let our own light shine, we unconsciously give other people permission to do the same. As we are liberated from our own fear, our presence automatically liberates others.

From *A Return to Love* by Marianne Williamson. Copyright © 1992 by Marianne Williamson. Reprinted with permission from HarperCollins Publishers.

Secondary Gains

Some of our clients may become anxious once their speech and language is improving or has been remediated. Clients may present with *secondary gains,* or psychological benefits derived from their challenge; for example, a PWS, a client with dysphonia, a client who has had articulation and/or language and literacy difficulties may have inadvertently benefitted from his speech and language disorder. The client's struggle may have provided an excuse not to socialize, speak out, read aloud in class, or to become complacent. When a clinician becomes aware of the possible benefits that the client may be deriving, albeit subconsciously, from his communication disorder, this sheds light for the clinician both diagnostically and therapeutically (Friedman, 2013).

Addressing Secondary Gains

Secondary gains may be a significant factor underlying the fear of success and may therefore block progress in therapy. One way of working on these maladaptive benefits is to have the client look through the following list of unconscious benefits and decide which ones apply:

- The responsibility that comes along with success could create significant anxiety for some individuals.
- For some people, feeling happy might set them apart from their family or peers, leaving them standing out, potentially evoking envy, and possibly feeling excluded and isolated. The fear of disconnection may override their desire for happiness.
- Giving up complacency and resigning oneself to helplessness.
- Having to give up and release the negative attention, which the communication disorder had perpetuated (Friedman, 2013).

- Some individuals may feel guilty for feeling happy when they compare their situation with those who are unhappy and less fortunate.

- When the external circumstances in our lives, such as career or relationship, are not aligned with our inner core beliefs (dissonance; i.e., when we believe we are not meant to be successful and happy), we may become anxious and frightened; there is an internal conflict (Ben-Shahar, 2010).

Reviewing the list would then prompt a discussion between client and clinician. Once there is awareness, the clinician may ask the client, "How might we handle this challenge and its unconscious benefits in a more adaptive and productive way? (Friedman, 2013). Cognitive behavioral therapy (see Chapter 8) may then be incorporated to help the client reframe or modify these subconscious beliefs.

For many of us, including our students and clients, the possibility of immediate happiness in the present is too terrifying, so we procrastinate. We search for happiness as some long-term goal in the far off future. We rationalize that we must prepare more, this is not a good time, we need to get all of our ducks in a row, and *then* we'll show up in the world (Box 3-9). Our students are so consumed with their academic and caseload responsibilities that they often believe happiness will only occur when their graduate training is completed. Ralph Waldo Emerson once said, "Life is a journey, not a destination."

Box 3-9

HAPPINESS IS A JOURNEY

We convince ourselves that life will be better after we get married, have a baby, then another. Then we're frustrated that the kids aren't old enough and we'll be more content when they are. After that, we're frustrated that we have teenagers to deal with. We'll certainly be happy when they're out of that stage.

We tell ourselves that our life will be complete when our spouse gets his or her act together, when we get a nicer car, are able to go on a nice vacation, when we retire.

The truth is, there's no better time to be happy than right now. If not now, when?

Your life will always be filled with challenges. It's best to admit this to yourself and decide to be happy anyway.

One of my favorite quotes comes from Alfred D. Souza. He said, "For a long time it had seemed to me that life was about to begin—real life. But there was always some obstacle in the way, something to be gotten through first, some unfinished business, time still to be served, or a debt to be paid. Then life would begin. At last it dawned on me that these obstacles were my life."

This perspective has helped me to see that there is no way to happiness. Happiness is the way. So, treasure every moment that you have and treasure it more because you shared it with someone special, special enough to spend your time with…and remember that time waits for no one.

(continued)

Box 3-9 (CONTINUED)

So, stop waiting until you finish school, until you go back to school, until you lose ten pounds, until you gain ten pounds, until you have kids, until your kids leave the house, until you start work, until you retire, until you get married, until you get divorced, until Friday night, until Sunday morning, until you get a new car or home, until your car or home is paid off, until spring, until summer, until fall, until winter, until you're off welfare, until the first or fifteenth, until your song comes on, until you've had a drink, until you've sobered up, until you die, until you're born again to decide that there is no better time than right now to be happy.

Happiness is a journey, not a destination.

As we get older, we are more guarded about letting in those moments of joy that come so naturally and spontaneously to children. We marvel at those instances, such as when a mother turns on music for her 18-month-old child who is in the middle of a tantrum, and he immediately switches to intense, unbridled joy and dances to the music.

Three ways to facilitate happiness in the moment are to listen to music, play with a pet, and/or interact with a child. Studies regarding rehabilitative care in nursing homes include bringing children to these facilities to sing and perform for the elderly (Seefeldt, 1987). If you have had the pleasure of seeing this occur, you may have noticed the immediate and spontaneous joy on the faces of the residents when they see these children. These incidents are when happiness is not on hold.

Ask Yourself

1. Where in your life can you give yourself permission to be human?

2. Bad things happen in every life. Think of a personal struggle and how you grew from it.

3. When a client sheds tears, notice your possible discomfort and where it comes from. Describe how you can learn to deal with it.

4. What shifts for you when you permit yourself to experience your full range of emotions?

5. Try comforting a friend when he is overwhelmed, upset, or anxious by applying what you have learned from this chapter. What was the result?

6. Write at least three times over the course of a day where you felt a happy feeling and you gave yourself permission to be in it and to let it run through your body.

7. Allow yourself to smile. Smiling is a powerful builder of self-esteem that enables us to deeply and completely feel our joy.

KEY CONCEPTS

- All human beings have positive and negative emotions.
- Feelings are neither good nor bad; they just *are*.
- We are not defective because we have painful emotions.
- As human beings and professionals, we must accept and process the full range of our emotions as well as those of our clients and their families.
- Empathy empowers, while sympathy disempowers.
- Our humanness makes us more alike than different.
- Suppression of painful emotion is counterproductive and harmful.
- As we honor our uncomfortable emotions, we create a space for positive emotions to flow inside of us.

- The more present we are, the more able we become to allow our families to go through their own grieving process.

- Without permission to be human, we stifle our own healing process as well as that of others.

- Fear of success occurs when we become anxious about realizing our goal—that is, when we fear success.

- Joining with the client means that we are able to sit with their painful and negative emotions without trying to fix or change them.

- The clinician must be prepared to engage in difficult conversations such as delivering bad news.

- The grief cycle includes five stages after loss: denial, anger, bargaining, depression, and acceptance.

- Possible reasons for experiencing fear of success are as follows:
  - The additional responsibility that comes with success
  - Not being part of a previous group of people
  - Giving up complacency
  - Secondary gains (e.g., negative attention)
  - Guilt for feeling happy and for achievement
  - Dissonance—when the external circumstances of our lives are not aligned with our beliefs about ourselves.

- Possible ways to encourage spontaneous happiness include the following:
  - Listen to music
  - Play with a pet
  - Interact with a child

REFERENCES

Ainsworth, S., & Fraser, J. (1988). *If your child stutters: A guide for parents* (3rd ed.). Memphis, TN: Speech Foundation of America.

Axline, R. (2014). Caring for others—and yourself. *The ASHA Leader.* Online only. doi:10.1044/leader.OV.19052014.np.

Ball, R. R. (2014). *Being with: Maybe this is what life is all about.* Bloomington, IN: Author House.

Bang, M. (1999). *When Sophie gets angry—really, really angry.* New York, NY: Blue Sky Press.

Ben-Shahar, T. (2010). *Foundations of positive psychology* [PowerPoint slides]. Retrieved from www.slideshare.net/dadalaolang/1504-01intro?ref=http://positivepsychologyprogram.com/harvard-positive-psychology-course

Boyd, C. (1997). *Happiness is a journey.* Retrieved from http://happinessisajourney.com.

Boyd, C. (2000). *Midnight muse.* n.p.: Moon Tiger Publishing.

Branden, N. (1995). *The six pillars of self-esteem: The definitive work on self-esteem by the leading pioneer in the field.* New York, NY: Bantam Books.

Brown, B. (2006). Shame resilience theory: A grounded theory study on women and shame. *Families in Society,* 87(1), 43–52.

Burns, D. D. (1999). *The feeling good handbook.* New York, NY: Plume.

Christensen, T. M., Skaggs, J. L., & Kleist, D. M. (1997). Traumatic brain injured families: Therapeutic considerations. *The Family Journal,* 5(4), 317–324.

Cohen, L. (1992). Anthem. On *The future.* New York, NY: Columbia.

Fialka, J. (1997). Advice to professionals who must "conference cases." *Dance of Partnership.* Retrieved from www.danceofpartnership.com/books.htm

Friedman, W. J. (2013). The benefits of suffering and the cost of well being: Secondary gains and losses [Web log post]. Mental Help. Retrieved from www.mentalhelp.net/blogs/the-benefits-of-suffering-and-the-costs-of-well-being-secondary-gains-and-losses/

Gottwald, S. R., & Starkweather, C. W. (1995). Fluency intervention for preschoolers and their families in the public schools. *Language, Speech, and Hearing Services in Schools, 26*(2), 117–126.

Hunting Pompon, R., Burns, M., & Kendall, D. L. (2015). Counseling the caregiver. *The ASHA Leader, 20*(7), 30–32. doi: 10.1044/leader.MIW.20072015.30. Retrieved from http://leader.pubs.asha.org/article.aspx?articleid=2389213.

Hutz, A. (2010). Leaning into discomfort. In M. Trotter-Mathison, J. M. Koch, S. Sanger, & T. M. Skovholt (Eds), *Voices from the field: Defining moments in counselor and therapist development.* Hoboken, NJ: Taylor & Francis, 2010.

Johnson, W., & Associates. (1959). *The onset of stuttering: Research findings and implications.* Minneapolis, MN: University of Minnesota.

Kimsey-House, H., Kimsey-House, K., Sandahl, P., & Whitworth, L. (2011). *Co-active coaching: Changing business, transforming lives.* Boston, MA: Nicholas Brealey.

Kübler-Ross, E. (1969). *On death and dying.* London, United Kingdom: Tavistock Publications.

Logan, K. J., & Yaruss, J. S. (1999). Helping parents address attitudinal and emotional factors with young children who stutter. *Contemporary Issues in Communication Science and Disorders, 26*(1), 69–81.

Merriam-Webster (n.d.). Empathy. *Merriam-Webster.* Retrieved from www.merriam-webster.com/dictionary/empathy.

Michallet, B., Le Dorze, G., & Tétreault, S. (2001). The needs of spouses caring for severely aphasic persons. *Aphasiology, 15*(8), 731–747.

Oriah Mountain Dreamer. (1999). *The invitation.* New York, New York: HarperCollins.

Riley, J. (2002). Counseling: An approach for speech-language pathologists. *Contemporary Issues in Communication Science and Disorders, 29*, 6-16.

Robinson, T. L., Jr. (2015). Handle with care. *The ASHA Leader, 20*(7), 24–25. doi: 10.1044/leader.OV.20072015.24.

Rogers, C. R. (1951). *Client-centered therapy: Its current practice, implications, and theory.* Boston, MA: Houghton Mifflin.

Rogers, F. M. (1968). What do you do with the mad that you feel? *PBS.* Retrieved from http://pbskids.org/rogers/songLyricsWhatDoYouDo.html

Seefeldt, C. (1987). The effects of preschoolers' visits to a nursing home. *The Gerontologist, 27*(2), 228–232.

Sheehan, J. G. (1970). *Stuttering: Research and therapy.* New York, NY: Harper & Row.

Stone, D., Patton, D., & Heen, S. (2010). *Difficult conversations.* London, United Kingdom: Penguin Books.

Thieda, K. (2014). Brené Brown on empathy vs. sympathy [Web log comment]. *Psychology Today.* Retrieved from www.psychologytoday.com/blog/partnering-in-mental-health/201408/bren-brown-empathy-vs-sympathy-0

Visser-Meily, A., Post, M., Gorter, J. W., Berlekom, S. B. V., Van Den Bos, T., & Lindeman, E. (2006). Rehabilitation of stroke patients needs a family-centered approach. *Disability and Rehabilitation, 28*(24), 1557–1561.

Wegner, D. M., Schneider, D. J., Carter, S. R., & White, T. L. (1987). Paradoxical effects of thought suppression. *Journal of Personality and Social Psychology, 53*(1), 5–13.

Whitworth, L. (2007). *Co-Active Coaching: New skills for coaching people toward success in work and life.* Mountain View, CA: Davies-Black Publishing.

Williamson, M. (1996). *A return to love: Reflections on the principles of a course of miracles.* San Francisco, CA: HarperOne.

Yaruss, J. S. (2010). Assessing quality of life in stuttering treatment outcomes research. *Journal of Fluency Disorders, 35*(3), 190–202.

Zebrowski, P. M., & Schum, R. L. (1993). Counseling parents of children who stutter. *American Journal of Speech-Language Pathology, 2*(2), 65–73.

4

Client as Expert

One's own self is well hidden from one's own self; of all mines of treasure, one's own is the last to be dug up.

—Friedrich Nietzsche

LEARNER OUTCOMES

After reading this chapter, the reader will be able to:

1. Describe the relevance of the person as "naturally creative, resourceful, and whole" (Kimsey-House, Kimsey-House, Sandahl, & Whitworth, 2011) to personal growth and to the counseling process for the speech-language pathologist and audiologist.

2. Identify and describe the two basic elements of the definition of self-esteem according to Branden.

3. Provide examples of how to build positive self-esteem.

4. Distinguish between counseling moments and teaching moments.

5. Describe the role of facilitating positive emotions in the clinical setting according to Fredrickson.

6. Describe some of the ways to empower children.

Recently, a former client of mine (BTA), now 19 years of age, returned to therapy after 7 years. She was originally diagnosed with language and learning difficulties.

According to the client, her mother encouraged her to return to therapy to address her "unclear speech" and "squeaky voice." The parent was concerned that her daughter's speech would make a "poor impression" at job interviews. During our initial discussion, she clearly expressed that she was not particularly interested in working on her speech. She added that her returning for remediation was her family's idea.

Stein-Rubin, C., & Adler, B. T. *Counseling in Communication Disorders: Facilitating the Therapeutic Rehabilitation* (pp 49-62).

During our initial discussion, my client expressed that she was not particularly interested in working on her speech; this had been her family's idea. She relayed that she has been feeling annoyed, frustrated, and angry that her family did not accept her and her "normal way of speaking." My client complained about being criticized frequently and feeling sad about it. I simply listened and then assured her that I would not impose my ideas on her and that we could continue to discuss the issues in terms of her best interests. She seemed surprised and pleased that I acknowledged her as a team member and validated her feelings. Following that exchange, I elicited several goals from my client specific to her speech-language improvement as well as communicating with her family. My client commented that she was pleased to feel part of the process rather than feeling imposed on and directed. This is an example of developing a partnership: respecting the client's needs and trusting that the individual will arrive at a positive solution.

Each one of us is an individual with the potential to improve and progress. Our work is most empowering to our clients when we view them and their families as "naturally creative, resourceful, and whole" (Kimsey-House et al., 2011)—or as the expert on their own lives. Likewise, when we as clinicians are able to see and recognize our own possibilities, as naturally creative, resourceful, and whole, we are then better able to support our clients to view themselves in this regard.

Our students and new clinicians often view their clients as broken, fragile, incomplete, and possibly incapable of managing their own obstacles without the clinician's help. Clinicians may view themselves as rescuers and fixers, which can damage the therapeutic relationship. To disregard the client's agenda and readiness is to impose change whether the client is ready for it or not. According to Rogers (1951) and Ouellette (2004), "unconditional positive regard," (Kimsey-House et al., 2011) or viewing the client and family as "naturally creative, resourceful, and whole," is another core condition for a powerful therapeutic relationship.

It is not our professional role to take control of another person's life. Recognizing the client's autonomy both improves client-clinician communication and alleviates the clinician's self-imposed pressure. The speech-language pathologist or audiologist must trust that the clients have the inherent resources, creativity, and wisdom to meet most of their own challenges. It is the clinician's job to create a safe and nonjudgmental space and to act as a catalyst—asking curious and powerful questions—for unlocking the client's potential. The clinician must believe that each person already carries the seeds for her own development and is therefore an expert in her own right (Botterill, 2011; Luterman, 2008; Ouellette, 2004; Riley, 2002; Whitworth, 2007).

In keeping with this perspective of the client as expert, the client has vital information to contribute, which may influence goal selection and achievement. To create the opportunity for clinicians and clients to work together in partnership, we remove the onus from the clinician to have to know everything, thus empowering the client. As such, we as clinicians remove our white coats, level the playing field, and work as a powerful team in collaboration with the client. On the basis of our clinical experience, we have used the term *reciprocal learning* to describe how our clients and students are often the vehicles for our own expanded learning. In other words, the clients or students trigger learning for us, as clinicians, supervisors, or instructors, and this is turn shapes our therapy or our teaching.

When we work with children, we also encourage the parents to tap into their own creativity and wisdom. The clinician acts as a guide to uncover the parents' resourcefulness. The objective is not to fix the child or make her dependent on the clinician; rather, the goal is to equip the parents with the confidence and tools to effectively raise their child (Zebrowski & Schum, 1993). Let's take a look at the relationships among Helen Keller, her teacher Anne Sullivan, and Helen's parents, who were not trained or guided to have an empowering relationship with their daughter (Luterman, 2008; Box 4-1).

Box 4-1

Helen's parents had been struggling to raise their atypical child, who became blind and deaf after a childhood illness and whose behavior was becoming out of control. Over time, they had been ineffective in managing her temper tantrums. When Helen was about 7 years old, her parents hired Anne Sullivan to be her teacher. Anne knew how to teach deaf children and had her own vision difficulties. To have greater control over Helen's behavior, Sullivan eventually needed to remove Helen from the main house and set up a separate living space for the two of them. In time, under Sullivan's care, Helen's communication improved. This occurred as soon as she made the connection that finger-spelling on her palm represented an object.

As extraordinary as this relationship may have been, Sullivan may not have trusted that the Kellers had the potential to be naturally creative, resourceful, and whole and, to some degree, an expert about their child. Anne Sullivan neglected to teach Helen's parents how to effectively parent her and to foster an expansive parent-child relationship. In retrospect, Sullivan rendered herself Helen's primary rescuer and fixer.

Ask Yourself

1. Have you ever given advice rather than holding the other person as naturally creative, resourceful, and whole?

2. Has anyone ever done this to you? How did it make you feel?

When we treat others and ourselves as naturally creative, resourceful, and whole, we increase our clients' self-esteem, that of their families, and our own. When we have healthy *self-esteem*, we trust our own minds; we view ourselves as competent and able, worthwhile, and deserving of happiness (Branden, 1995). To summarize Branden's theory, self-esteem has two parts: *self-efficacy/competence* and *worthiness*.

SELF-EFFICACY AND COMPETENCE

According to Branden (1995), self-efficacy is when we "trust in our processes—and as a consequence, we expect success for our efforts." In contrast, when we feel insecure and uncertain about our choices, we question ourselves, expect to fail, and may beat ourselves up for the choices we did or did not make. This cycle may occur in everyday life and in the therapeutic setting. An example of everyday life is given in Box 4-2.

BOX 4-2

I (CSR) recall a day in the early '70s that my father, a structural engineer, received the dreaded pink slip. Given his competence and expertise, he was quickly hired by another engineering firm. After a week or two, overwhelmed by the demands of the new job, he decided to quit. The next day, my father informed his boss that he did not have the training and expertise required to manage his new position. Even though my father lacked belief in himself, his boss believed in my father's inherent capacity and asked him not to quit. With the proper encouragement, my father relaxed, and the demands of his new position started to feel more natural to him. He quickly moved up the ranks to become head of the department, a job that proved rewarding and fulfilling until the day he retired.

The only way to feel secure about our choices is to be an active agent in our own lives. Part of self-efficacy is clarifying for ourselves what we don't know and having the resourcefulness and courage to ask for the appropriate help. Self-reliance doesn't mean never reaching out to others; in fact, some of us must seek help to tap into innate resourcefulness and creativity. Seeking help requires self-trust in and courage to ask. We must also trust in those who support us.

Furthermore, self-trust transcends confidence in specific skills like engineering, math, or art. It is a belief that our own resources, creativity, logic, and emotional intelligence will allow us to handle whatever life throws our way. Inevitably, we'll make mistakes, but we need not lose ourselves because of them.

A significant part of self-esteem or confidence in our competence is having the willingness not to need to be perfect. Ben-Shahar (2010) talks about the importance of making mistakes as part of learning and growing, emphasizing that growing is about not being afraid to falter; rather it means putting ourselves on the line, falling, and getting up. To sum up this outlook, Ben-Shahar coined the phrase, "Learn to fail, or fail to learn."

Because we must make mistakes to learn, we must open ourselves up to all types of feedback so that we may continue to grow. No one enjoys hearing feedback that is less than positive. Our students often want to impress supervisors and instructors and to do everything "perfectly." Yet this point of view leads to a narrow perception of the circumstance and of the *self*. The reality is that we may use our mistakes as opportunities for personal and professional growth and may need to change our perspective about another's honest feedback.

We may see the effects of one not trusting in one's competence in the therapeutic setting. Parents often express a range of feelings, including helplessness, insecurity, uncertainty, feeling overwhelmed, guilt, anger, blame, and anxiety. Some or all of these emotions may occur in the early days of therapy. To facilitate competence in parents, it is critical for the clinician to listen to the parents' feelings empathically and nonjudgmentally. The clinician may then name the feeling that she hears beneath the words. As noted in Chapter 3, allowing individuals to process their emotions (and avoid jumping into fixing mode) increases their self-esteem. These opportunities for the clinician to reflect on the client or family member's feelings have been referred to as *counseling moments*.

Luterman (2006) distinguishes between *teaching moments* and *counseling moments*. The purpose of the former is to deliver information. Although a client's comment may sound as if she is asking for technical knowledge (teaching moment), hearing the feeling (counseling moment) may be more appropriate and effective for her healing at that point in time. Often, the client is not at the point to process technical knowledge. For example, the parent who asks, "What causes stuttering?" may really be asking, "What did I do to cause my child's stuttering?" In this case, the clinician may need to address the parent's guilt over her child's struggle. To open that dialogue, the clinician might then say, "What do you know about the causes of stuttering?" According to Luterman, the most important ingredient in counseling is having the ability to distinguish between teachable and counseling moments; effective counseling is composed of a combination of the two (Luterman, 2006, 2008).

The following are examples of how clinicians may build family members' self-esteem and competence when facing their child's communication challenge:

Parent: I think I came here too late.

Clinician: From what you have said, you discovered your child's difficulty recently. It sounds like you're beating yourself up for something that you didn't even know.

Another response may apply: You are actually here at the right stage of your child's development. Intervention will be more effective at this current stage.

Parent: I just want my child to be like everyone else, I want my child to be regular.

Clinician: I hear that you may be feeling frustrated and concerned about how your child will fit in with the other children. This is a common worry for parents. Let's start out by recognizing your child's strengths.

Parent: Will my daughter be okay? Will she ever be able to take care of herself or have a career?

Clinician: It sounds as if you are very worried about your daughter and her future. We plan to work together step by step. As you see the progress, the anxiety is likely to diminish.

Parent: I'm just not sure what to do, what the next step is—I'm so confused.

Clinician: This can definitely be overwhelming, and there is no question it can be confusing. I will do my best to answer your questions and clarify whatever is confusing to you. Please write down questions when you leave here so that we can go over them when you return. We can take this one step at a time.

When we acknowledge and name what parents may be feeling, they feel heard, more secure, less isolated, more connected, and part of a team. This type of conversation builds their sense of competence. Following the validation of the parents' emotions, we are then able to move onto refocusing the conversation to what's working and to the child's and the family's strengths. We often suggest to the parent that we are going to turn from the past and focus on what we may all do in the present to help their child. The more we support parents to stay present, the calmer and more in control they seem to feel. That said, if self-esteem issues are complicated, Robinson (2015) suggested working with the parents, classroom teacher, school counselor, and/or psychologist as a team in the process.

Ask Yourself

1. Name a time in your life when you felt competent enough to handle a difficult situation. What did it require of you to handle it?

2. Where in your life have you tried to be "perfect," and how would allowing yourself to make mistakes have changed the outcome?

3. What is a challenging question that a parent may have asked you, and what was your answer?

Self-Fulfilling Prophecy

Research in the areas of business and education indicates that when expectations of students or employees are held high, they perform better (Buckingham & Clifton, 2001). The reverse is also true; treating an individual as if she is incapable diminishes her ability to perform. Therefore, a person who holds herself as naturally creative, resourceful, and whole may create a *self-fulfilling prophecy*, a prediction that directly or indirectly brings about positive reinforcement between the belief and the believer. In contrast, a person who does not hold herself that way may create a negative self-fulfilling prophecy.

In the arena of assessment and therapy, holding a client and family member to high expectations means acknowledging them as naturally creative, resourceful, and whole. Studies have shown that clients and families will return to therapy when the clinician treats them with respect and shows confidence in them from the initial stages of an interview. In addition, these clients demonstrate more consistency and make better long-term progress (Miller & Rollnick, 2012).

Acting As If

Acting as if has been discussed in both popular and psychological literature. It is an important part of achieving a positive self-fulfilling prophecy. By *acting as if*, we mean if you want to be calm, act calm. If you want to be happy, act happy. Research indicates that when you smile, it tricks your brain into thinking you are happy. This lifts our endorphin levels (happiness hormones), and we actually feel happier. Feeling happier, in turn, impacts how we view ourselves and consequently how others view us. This creates a cycle of happiness, which may become contagious in our interactions with others.

Broaden-and-Build Theory

According to Barbara Fredrickson and her *broaden-and-build theory* (2004), positive emotions actually open our minds to notice positivity around us. When exposed to positive emotions, our minds expand, and we are more likely to see the broader picture—that's the broaden part. As a result of this awareness, we become better able to problem solve, be more creative, and more resourceful—that's the build part.

On the other hand, when we experience negative emotions, it causes our mind to shrink and to narrow, and this limits our possibilities in terms of innovation, creativity, resourcefulness, and problem solving. We move into a *fight-or-flight* reaction or *survival mode* to just simply get through the experience, unscathed, rather than to open ourselves up to possibilities (Fredrickson, 2001).

Lyubomirsky, King, and Diener (2005) found that success makes people happy; however, positive affect also engenders success. The implications for the speech-language pathologist and audiologist in this regard are significant. Sharp (2011) notes that the integration of positive emotions into therapy will enhance therapeutic performance and outcomes. These results may be seen in client engagement, tendency to complete carryover assignments, and ability to generalize therapeutic concepts.

As speech-language pathology and audiology clinicians, we deal with clients who make the assumption that they'll be happy once they reach their therapeutic goals (see Chapter 3). Yet, what if the process of reaching the goals falls below the client's expectations? What if the process was arduous and had many ups and downs? What if the client didn't quite reach her goals in the end?

Intervention is a process that takes time. It does not always move in a linear and forward direction. Clients may regress and become frustrated along the path. The clinician's role is to examine what is working and to build on it with the client. We may need to recognize whether a therapeutic technique is suitable for the client. We may need to break it down into smaller pieces, simplify the steps, or change the method. While the clinician makes the appropriate adjustments in treatment, it is essential to maintain a positive attitude and provide emotional support.

If clients experience positive emotions as, perhaps, an implicit goal, their "success" is then more likely to follow. At the same time, it is also quite possible that positive emotions are not just experienced as a result of success. Positive emotions and attitudes may become catalysts for the client to reach her goals (Sharp, 2011).

In terms of the clinician working on *self* to reach professional goals, it is important to note that the following principles of positivity, adapted from Sharp (2011), may contribute to the clinician and client achieving success:

- Positive psychology directly encourages and is built on connectedness and positive relationships.
- Maintaining positive emotion will boost self-esteem, self-respect, learning, and assertiveness.
- A positive focus emphasizes developing strengths.
- Positivity boosts resilience and enhances coping abilities.

We have both found that we tend to create warm and nurturing classroom environments conducive to learning. When a student is in this type of space, there is an increase in positive emotions, and negative emotions such as anxiety diminish. Research cited by Fredrickson (2004) indicates that when both children and adults are exposed to positive emotions, such as memorable experiences or in positive films, they perform better on subsequent tasks.

Ask Yourself

1. What does self-fulfilling prophecy mean to you?

2. When have you *acted as if* and what was the impact of this on you and others?

3. How has experiencing positive emotions connected to success in your life?

WORTHINESS

The second part of the definition of self-esteem, *worthiness*, is about self-respect; it means believing in one's own self-worth and right to happiness. When we consider the phrase *naturally creative, resourceful, and whole*, worthiness speaks to the last word—*whole*. To achieve a sense of worthiness, we must learn to accept our virtues as well as our limitations, and, as discussed in Chapter 3, to love ourselves regardless of our shortcomings.

All relationships, between adults or parent–child, may suffer if a sense of worthiness is missing. Unfortunately, we often seek to change others, which implies to the other person that who they are is not good enough. Change requires the complete acceptance, or unconditional positive regard (Rogers, 1951), of the other individual. In an empowered relationship, we accept all parts of the other person, just as we would want to be accepted. When we love all of someone, including her shortcomings, we experience a deeper and more rewarding love. Parents of children with disabilities are often inspiring examples of that kind of love—they get to experience that the whole is greater than the sum of its parts.

Once individuals recognize that they are fully accepted, they may then be open to engaging in the process of change. This process must be conducted with the utmost sensitivity. To love and accept ourselves, which is the key to loving and accepting others, we must develop our *inner core values*, or the way we perceive ourselves in relation to the universe. From a young age, we develop these values unconsciously. For example, if we grew up with parents who insisted that we not draw attention to ourselves, that we choose a safe and practical career, and that we keep a low personal profile, we internalize those values and make them an integral part of our personal and world view (Box 4-3).

Box 4-3

I (CSR) have an adult female client who came to me seeking help with her public speaking ability. The reality was that her oral communication skills were quite good, although she did not believe that this was the case. The client seemed to have a misperception of her true abilities and this contributed to her core beliefs about herself and her diminished attempts to "speak up."

She recently began her first full-time position and noted that her fears of speaking up, both one-on-one and at meetings, stemmed from a feeling that, when expressing herself, she would not measure up to other people's expectations. Although she had many relevant ideas and experiences to share, she was fearful that she would disappoint in her delivery. In a sense, she felt "trapped or caged" because she didn't feel free to completely relay her true thoughts, ideas, and experiences. Unless the client changed her own worldview of who she was in an interpersonal communication situation, her lack of confidence in her speaking skills were likely to continue.

We worked with a tape recorder, and as she listened, she wrote a list of all the aspects of her communication that she liked; there were many. The client came to the conclusion that she was being "too hard on herself" and that she sounded far better than the way that she had perceived herself. She soon began taking risks, speaking up and expressing herself more authentically. This further reinforced her new core value and her image of herself as a competent communicator.

Our job is to help our clients improve their communicative competence. This is often intertwined with their limiting beliefs, defeatist attitudes, inaccurate assumptions, and distorted core beliefs. Sometimes this does not involve direct speech work; rather, it involves looking at the whole human being, seeing them as capable, and then helping them to see themselves a bit differently. We act as a catalyst to bring out what our clients may truly be capable of doing—to assist them to become experts on their lives.

Empowering Children

Children are also naturally creative, resourceful, and whole and deserve to feel worthy. When raising my (BTA) children in the late '60s to early '70s, I began to follow the teachings of the psychologist Dr. Haim Ginott, who often talked about giving children some choices that would allow them to take responsibility. It would be the parent, however, who would set up the choices. For instance, at dinnertime, if the child didn't want her food, the parent could divide the food on her plate, and the child could then choose to eat the food from whichever side of the plate she wanted. "You're in charge of that," the parent would say. Most times children would make a selection and follow through. Struggling at mealtime was reduced, and children were reported to feel much happier being part of making decisions.

This one idea set me on a path of following this same principle in my therapy room and one that, during supervision, I encouraged student-clinicians to follow. Clinicians encourage non-compliant children to be the bosses for the session by choosing the activity they would like to do first. For example, I might place three labeled sticky notes on a table that read as follows: "Read together," "Computer time," and "Notebook practice." The child then chooses the order of the activities. This has worked for an endless number of disinterested children, who then came to the therapy room excited and cooperative. This one small change provided the opportunity for the children to be active in the process, to have increased confidence and self-esteem, and to feel worthy.

Several books have been inspired by the principles and teachings of Dr. Haim Ginott, including works by Drs. Faber and Mazlish (2012), beginning with their book, *How to Talk So Kids Will Listen and Listen So Kids Will Talk*. Their books focused on the way parents and teachers need to listen and learn how to reflect back their children's message. When we respond with questions, choices, options, and acknowledgment, children become active agents, whether at home, school, or in our therapy rooms (Box 4-4).

Box 4-4

My (BTA) friend shared a story about her 11-year-old granddaughter, who is quite bright and doing well in school. The difficulty was that she has always avoided engaging in conversations with her parents that may have required her to be more aware of her behavior. Whenever her parents attempted to talk with her about their observations related to schoolwork, family chores, sibling rivalry, and so on, she would become defensive and upset. All attempts turned into lectures and crying, rather than supportive talks. When she began to display some disorganization about her schoolwork, her parents wanted to teach her how to be more organized and efficient. Fortunately, they decided not to impose change by attempting to talk about it. Instead, they were encouraged to write a letter to her expressing their desire to support her with her work and to set up a time to brainstorm ideas together as a team. The daughter agreed to meet with her parents to work though her organizational difficulties.

(continued)

BOX 4-4 (CONTINUED)

By recognizing their daughter's difficulty and sensitivity with reflective conversations, these parents chose a non-confrontational alternative for change. They provided an opportunity for their child to make her own choice and for them to work together. They empowered her in the relationship and made her feel worthy.

When we provide children with choices, we are treating them with respect. When children are treated with respect, they learn to treat others with respect. As they gain self-esteem and confidence because they are viewed in this light, they are willing to be more cooperative. It becomes the parent's and the clinician's job to act as catalysts and models to bring out the child's ability to be in partnership and to be part of the learning process (Box 4-5).

BOX 4-5

I (BTA) recall a phone call from a parent of a 5-year-old client. The child was being bullied verbally at day camp, and out of frustration, he hit the bullies. Even though his mother agreed that the bullies were saying upsetting things, she didn't want her son to react with physical violence. She tried to coach him on what to say in response to the teasing and reprimanded him for hitting.

Unfortunately, the situation just kept getting worse. She called me for some guidance. I encouraged the mother to ask her son if he thought the insults were true. If he did, then by asking him simple logical questions, she could help him to see that, in fact, the bullies' words were exaggerations. If he said that he did not think the insults were true, they could skip that step and move right into discussing what would be acceptable behavior for both him and the other children.

By allowing him to answer questions, rather than just telling him what to think, he would not only understand, he would also be able verbalize his understanding of what was true and what was exaggerated. Likewise, the mother would assist her son in arriving at a solution without reprimanding him for his understandable reactions. He would become part of the solution rather than part of the problem. I encouraged the mother to acknowledge her son as naturally creative, resourceful, and whole; to guide him toward acceptable reactions; and to build his self-esteem. I also advised her to speak with the director of the camp about better managing the bullies.

CONCLUSION

Many believe that self-esteem is unchangeable; however, positive psychologists and cognitive behavioral therapists have shown otherwise (Ben-Shahar, 2010; Branden, 1995). Our years in the field have taught us that people can change. Although we've seen many people sabotage their own success, in part because their core value is that people can't change, we have also seen people raise their self-esteem.

Some of our clients have expressed their feelings of being overwhelmed, embarrassed, and angered about their learning weaknesses and speech and language difficulties. These clients started out believing that they would never achieve success, always remain behind, and always be different from the other students. They were so beaten down—by their struggles and by the way that others treated them—that they began to believe they weren't worthy of success. During their time in therapy, as we witnessed their progress, we also saw a change in attitude. Our clients' grades and social connections improved. Several of them applied to schools that specialized in their artistic abilities.

As clinicians and supervisors, we must subscribe to the core value of the human capacity for change. We must have faith in the inherent competence and resourcefulness of individuals and families to alter the way they view themselves and, subsequently, the way they behave. We believe that everyone is naturally creative, resourceful, and whole. We, as clinicians, must examine our unique styles, gifts, and resources, as well as those of our clients, to bring these to the therapeutic relationship. We must work on gaining greater access to those characteristics, build a strengths-based vocabulary, and trust in our natural abilities to connect with people.

Ask Yourself

1. What shifts for you as clinician or clinical supervisor when you hold yourself as naturally creative, resourceful, and whole?

2. How does your paradigm shift when you trust in your client's inherent wisdom?

3. What changes for you when you trust in your ability to connect with people?

4. Self-Esteem:

   a. What are your sources of self-esteem?

b. How can you develop self-esteem in yourself and in others?

c. In which areas do you have self-esteem?

d. In which areas would you like to develop greater self-esteem (Ben-Shahar, 2010)?

KEY CONCEPTS

- Believing that everyone is naturally creative, resourceful, and whole corresponds to unconditional positive regard as one of Carl Rogers's key ingredients for a successful counseling relationship.
- When we hold ourselves as naturally creative, resourceful, and whole, we trust in the inherent wisdom and strength of the human spirit.
- A person who sees herself as naturally creative, resourceful, and whole creates a self-fulfilling prophecy for success.
- A negative self-fulfilling prophecy generates a vicious cycle, affecting how we behave and how we interact with others.
- A negative self-fulfilling prophecy decreases self-esteem.
- Self-esteem, according to Branden, comprises two parts: self-efficacy (competence) and worthiness.
- Barbara Fredrickson developed the *broaden-and-build theory*, which explains the role of positive emotions in achieving success.
- Empower children by providing choices.

REFERENCES

Ben-Shahar, T. (2010). *Foundations of positive psychology* [PowerPoint slides]. Retrieved from www.slideshare.net/dadalaolang/1504-01intro?ref=http://positivepsychologyprogram.com/harvard-positive-psychology-course.

Botterill, W. (2011). Developing the therapeutic relationship: From "expert" professional to "expert" person who stutters. *Journal of Fluency Disorders, 36*(3), 158–173.

Branden, N. (1995). *The six pillars of self-esteem: The definitive work on self-esteem by the leading pioneer in the field.* New York, NY: Bantam Books.

Buckingham, M., & Clifton, D. O. (2001). *Now, discover your strengths.* New York, NY: Simon & Schuster.

Faber, A., & Mazlish, E. (2012). *How to talk so kids will listen & so kids will talk.* New York, NY: Simon and Schuster.

Fredrickson, B. L. (2001). The role of positive emotions in positive psychology: The broaden-and-build theory of positive emotions. *American Psychologist, 56*(3), 218–226.

Fredrickson, B. L. (2004). The broaden-and-build theory of positive emotions. *Philosophical Transactions of the Royal Society of London, Series B: Biological Sciences, 359,* 1367–1378.

Kimsey-House, H., Kimsey-House, K., Sandahl, P., & Whitworth, L. (2011). *Co-active coaching: Changing business, transforming lives.* Boston, MA: Nicholas Brealey.

Luterman, D. (2006). *Children with hearing loss: A family guide.* Sedona, AZ: Auricle Ink.

Luterman, D. (2008). *Counseling persons with communication disorders and their families* (5th ed.). Austin, TX: Pro-Ed.

Lyubomirsky, S., King, L., & Diener, E. (2005). The benefits of frequent positive affect: Does happiness lead to success? *Psychological Bulletin, 131*(6), 803–855.

Miller, W. R., & Rollnick, S. (2012). *Motivational interviewing: Helping people change.* New York, NY: Guilford Press.

Ouellette, S. E. (2004). Clinical issues: Applications of solution-focused concepts to the practice of speech-language pathology. *SIG 1 Perspectives on Language Learning and Education, 11*(1), 8–14.

Riley, J. (2002). Counseling: An approach for speech-language pathologists. *Contemporary Issues in Communication Science and Disorders, 29,* 6–16.

Robinson Jr., T. L. (2015). Handle with care. *The ASHA Leader, 20*(7), 24–25. doi: 10.1044/leader.OV.20072015.24.

Rogers, C. R. (1951). *Client-centered therapy: Its current practice, implications, and theory.* Boston, MA: Houghton Mifflin.

Sharp, T. (2011). The primacy of positivity—applications in a coaching context. *Coaching: An International Journal of Theory, Research and Practice, 4*(1), 42–49.

Whitworth, L. (2007). *Co-active coaching: New skills for coaching people toward success in work and life.* Mountain View, CA: Davies-Black.

Zebrowski, P. M., & Schum, R.L. (1993). Counseling parents of children who stutter. *American Journal of Speech-Language Pathology, 2*(2), 65–73.

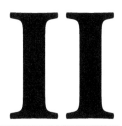

Essential Skills

- Chapter 5: Deep Listening
- Chapter 6: Language: The Power of Words
- Chapter 7: Developing Strengths
- Chapter 8: Raising Resilience

Once we have developed and established "knowing ourselves" and have practiced the three powerful perspectives, we may explore the skills needed to facilitate the therapeutic relationship and change. As clinicians skillfully trained in the methods needed specific to communication disorders, we must not make assumptions about our own ability to listen to others. We must not assume that we know how to use our words effectively. We often do not recognize our own strengths and resilience and may not know how to build these in our clients. By working on these skills within ourselves, we become the model for our students and clients and may better understand their struggles with change.

5

Deep Listening

Put your ear down close to your soul and listen hard.

—Anne Sexton

LEARNER OUTCOMES

After reading this chapter, the reader will be able to:

1. Identify the strengths and pitfalls of one's listening.
2. Describe the importance and relationship of deep listening to counseling for the speech-language pathologist and audiologist.
3. Explain the three levels of listening according to Kimsey-House, Kimsey-House, Sandahl, and Whitworth.
4. Cite, explain, and learn how to overcome the multiple roadblocks to effective listening.
5. Describe the role of silence in counseling for speech-language pathologists and audiologists.
6. Describe how we, as speech-language and hearing clinicians, train parents to listen to their children.

One of my (CSR) adult clients struggled with shyness and social pragmatic skills. She was uncomfortable in conversations, claiming that she never knew how to initiate one, how to gain access to a conversation, or maintain one. The client especially dreaded group social events such as parties. Although many individuals feel somewhat awkward or reticent about attending a party, this client was terrified. She compared herself with other outgoing and vivacious women who all seemed confident and excited about conversing. The client said that she longed to be like them, but when she attempted to imitate their behavior, she felt foolish and disingenuous.

Stein-Rubin, C., & Adler, B. T. *Counseling in Communication Disorders: Facilitating the Therapeutic Rehabilitation* (pp 65-83). © 2017 Taylor & Francis Group.

My client further noted that she preferred listening to talking. We worked together to create a plan as to how she might use her listening to be herself and to facilitate conversing with others. Together, we reviewed some principles of listening such as reflecting back, paraphrasing, and clarifying, which you will see in this chapter. My client returned from a dreaded party in a state of exuberance. She relayed how she had had several conversations with different people and added that the individuals all opened up and spoke to her for quite some time. She and two others exchanged phone numbers to keep in touch. My client began to realize that she was a talented listener, owned this strength, and began using it in a variety of new ways and settings.

When was the last time someone listened to you—stopping whatever he was doing to make you his sole focus and asking you deep reflective questions? Who was that person? Was it a favorite relative from your childhood—a parent, grandparent, aunt, or uncle? Think about what made that person so special. Chances are, he listened to you; he was genuinely curious about your thoughts and your life. What a powerful and rare gift! To feel heard is healing and transformative.

When we consider the act of communication, we might assume that speaking is of the utmost importance; however, the greatest power lies in listening. The skill of empathic and effective listening is invaluable. As you will see in Chapters 5 and 6, listening often determines the way we speak and our responses determine how the other person listens to and hears us. We must be aware of the reciprocal relationship between our listening and speaking to achieve optimal communication.

It is critical that we are attentive to understanding the speaker's words and perspective. It may be tempting for us to jump in with a solution to their problem, to complete their thought, or to express a professional opinion before we have gained a clear understanding of the situation, whether personal or professional. Once we understand the speaker's message, the listener may offer suggestions. This makes it more likely that the speaker will follow through on the listener's suggestions and own their behavior (Ouellette, 2004).

While listening may come naturally to some people, many of us lack polished listening skills. Fortunately, we can develop and hone these skills through consistent awareness, application of the tools in this chapter, and practice. These skills are essential for our professional growth and effective communication.

Ask Yourself

Write about a time when someone truly listened to you. How did it feel?

LISTENING AND THE HELPING PROFESSIONS

As health care professionals, our willingness and ability to listen empathically significantly affects our work. According to David Luterman (2008), "Listening is the gateway to counseling." As part of the foundation of the therapeutic relationship, effective listening transcends what our ears hear. To preserve the client's agenda, to truly hear what he needs, we must also use our eyes and hearts to pay him the deepest possible attention (Maggiani, 2009). "The professional sets aside his agenda in order to engage in deep selfless listening to the client" (Luterman, 2008). As helping professionals, listening empathically may be one of the greatest gifts we can give our clients.

As speech-language pathologists we tend to orient toward *active listening*, which refers to the postures and gestures of listening (Shafir, 2003). However, how much authentic and empathic listening do we actually incorporate into our communication with clients and students? Sometimes we concentrate so hard on looking as if we are listening that we may forget to listen.

The poem in Box 5-1 illustrates the common human desire to be heard.

Box 5-1

ON LISTENING

When I ask you to listen to me and you start giving advice, you have not done what I asked.

When I ask you to listen to me and you begin to tell me why I shouldn't feel that way, you are trampling on my feelings.

When I ask you to listen to me and you feel you have to do something to solve my problem, you have failed me, strange as that may seem.

Listen! All I asked was that you listen; not talk or do—just hear me.

And I can do for myself. I'm not helpless. Maybe discouraged and faltering, but not helpless.

When you do something for me that I can and need to do for myself, you contribute to my fear and feelings of inadequacy.

But, when you accept as a simple fact that I do feel what I feel, no matter how irrational, then I can quit trying to convince you and can get about the business of understanding what's behind this irrational feeling. And when that's clear, the answers are obvious and I don't need advice.

Irrational feelings make sense when we understand what's behind them.

So please listen and just hear me. And, if you want to talk, wait a minute for your turn. And I will listen to you.

Reprinted with permission from Ralph Roughton.

LEARN ABOUT YOUR LISTENING

When our students first learn about listening, they are often resistant. "Well, this is how all of my friends and family communicate," they say. "No one ever finishes speaking before someone else jumps in." They'll tell us that the listening skills we attempt to teach them feel unnatural. Our response to their resistance is that it is common to assume that our listening habits are just fine, typical, and acceptable, until we learn how much better they could be.

In her book *The Zen of Listening* (2003), Rebecca Shafir explains how to engage in deep empathic listening. Her experience as a speech-language pathologist and clinical supervisor in hospitals revealed that it's rare for health care professionals to listen deeply to clients and their families, or even to one another. She attributes her own professional burnout to a lack of effective listening in her workplace. We encourage you to complete Shafir's Listening Survey in Box 5-2 to examine your own listening skills. Her survey will help you discover what type of listener you are. We also recommend retaking the survey after you have focused on your listening skills for comparative purposes.

Box 5-2

Self knowledge is the first step toward self-improvement. Let's take a look at how well you listen today. This pretest will also make you aware of a wide spectrum of listening behaviors we intend to discuss. Carefully consider each question and indicate whether or not you consistently demonstrate each behavior. Then check your responses with the answer key on the next page and total your score.

Do you:

1. Think about what *you* are going to say while the speaker is talking?
   ☐ Yes, consistently   ☐ No, almost never   ☐ Sometimes

2. Tune out people who say things you don't agree with or don't want to hear?
   ☐ Yes, consistently   ☐ No, almost never   ☐ Sometimes

3. Learn something from each person you meet, even if it is ever so slight?
   ☐ Yes, consistently   ☐ No, almost never   ☐ Sometimes

4. Keep eye contact with the person who is speaking?
   ☐ Yes, consistently   ☐ No, almost never   ☐ Sometimes

5. Become self-conscious in one-to-one or small group conversations?
   ☐ Yes, consistently   ☐ No, almost never   ☐ Sometimes

6. Often interrupt the speaker?
   ☐ Yes, consistently   ☐ No, almost never   ☐ Sometimes

7. Fall asleep or daydream during meetings or presentations?
   ☐ Yes, consistently   ☐ No, almost never   ☐ Sometimes

8. Restate instructions or messages to be sure you understood correctly?
   ☐ Yes, consistently   ☐ No, almost never   ☐ Sometimes

9. Allow the speaker to vent negative feelings towards you without becoming defensive or physically tense?
   ☐ Yes, consistently   ☐ No, almost never   ☐ Sometimes

10. Listen for the meaning behind the speaker's words through gestures and facial expressions?
    ☐ Yes, consistently   ☐ No, almost never   ☐ Sometimes

(continued)

Box 5-2 (CONTINUED)

11. Feel frustrated or impatient when communicating with persons from other cultures?
☐ Yes, consistently ☐ No, almost never ☐ Sometimes

12. Inquire about the meaning of unfamiliar words or jargon?
☐ Yes, consistently ☐ No, almost never ☐ Sometimes

13. Give the appearance of listening when you are not?
☐ Yes, consistently ☐ No, almost never ☐ Sometimes

14. Listen to the speaker without judging or criticizing?
☐ Yes, consistently ☐ No, almost never ☐ Sometimes

15. Start giving advice before you are asked?
☐ Yes, consistently ☐ No, almost never ☐ Sometimes

16. Ramble on before getting to the point?
☐ Yes, consistently ☐ No, almost never ☐ Sometimes

17. Take notes when necessary to help you remember?
☐ Yes, consistently ☐ No, almost never ☐ Sometimes

18. Consider the state of the person you are talking to (nervous, rushed, hearing impaired, etc.)?
☐ Yes, consistently ☐ No, almost never ☐ Sometimes

19. Let a speaker's physical appearance or mannerisms distract you from listening?
☐ Yes, consistently ☐ No, almost never ☐ Sometimes

20. Remember a person's name after you have been introduced?
☐ Yes, consistently ☐ No, almost never ☐ Sometimes

21. Assume you know what the speaker is going to say and stop listening?
☐ Yes, consistently ☐ No, almost never ☐ Sometimes

22. Feel uncomfortable allowing silence between you and your conversation partner?
☐ Yes, consistently ☐ No, almost never ☐ Sometimes

23. Ask for feedback to make sure you are getting across to the other person?
☐ Yes, consistently ☐ No, almost never ☐ Sometimes

24. Preface your statements with unflattering remarks about yourself?
☐ Yes, consistently ☐ No, almost never ☐ Sometimes

25. Think more about building warm working relationships with team members and customers than about bringing in revenue?
☐ Yes, consistently ☐ No, almost never ☐ Sometimes

(continued)

Box 5-2 (CONTINUED)

Scoring: Compare your answers with those on the chart below. For every answer that matches the key, give yourself one point. If you answered "Sometimes" to any of the questions, score half a point. Total the number of points.

```
1 N   6 N   11 N   16 N   21 N
2 N   7 N   12 Y   17 Y   22 N
3 Y   8 Y   13 N   18 Y   23 Y
4 Y   9 Y   14 Y   19 N   24 N
5 N   10 Y  15 N   20 Y   25 Y
```

Total points: _____

If you scored 21 or more points, congratulations! Continue to read on and reinforce what you already are doing well. Note which areas could use further improvement. Are there any listening behaviors that require more consistency?...Good listeners can fine-tune listening under stress...and help others listen better.

A score of 16 to 20 suggests that you usually absorb most of the main ideas, but often miss a good portion of the rest of the message due to difficulties with sustaining attention. You may feel detached from the speaker and start thinking about other things or about what you are going to say next. Students who score at this level frequently comment that rechecking details is often needed...Examine typical response styles...that may prevent you from receiving that extra information.

If you scored between 10 and 15 points, you may be focusing more on your own agenda than the speaker's needs. You easily become distracted and perceive listening as a task. Perhaps personal biases get in the way of fully understanding the speaker...

Those of you who scored fewer than 9 points will notice the most dramatic improvement in your communication by applying the suggestions given in this book. Most of the time you experience listening as a boring activity. You might complain often that your memory is poor and feel great frustration when trying to retain information from presentations and succeed in a classroom situation.

If you answered "Sometimes" to many questions, then obviously you are a sometimes listener. Chances are your ability to concentrate and/or you are a highly critical individual and quick to judge whether a listening opportunity is worthwhile. However, there have been times when you have experienced the satisfaction of being fully absorbed in what someone has to say. Imagine how successful and effective you could be if you would let yourself experience that sense of total absorption in every listening opportunity.

Reprinted with permission from Shafir, R. Z. (2003). *The Zen of listening: Mindful communication in the age of distraction.* Wheaton, IL: Quest Books.

Many of the graduate students in the Therapeutic Relationship course we teach at Brooklyn College in New York are surprised when they see the results of their survey. Some become somewhat defensive, noting that the survey did not reflect the kind of listener they think they are. They tell us, "I always thought I was such a good listener," or "I can listen and do other things at the same time." Like many of us, they take their listening abilities for granted. Our students also observe that their listening changes with different settings and communication partners. For example, they comment that they might listen more intently in a more professional setting than they would with their family and peers. The Listening Survey is a productive first step to help our students recognize and clarify the nature of their listening. The next step is to learn about the different levels of listening.

Three Levels of Listening

The Co-Active Coaching model (Kimsey-House, Kimsey-House, Sandahl, & Whitworth, 2011) identifies three different levels of listening. Mastering all the levels, particularly II and III, will allow you to be more present and confident during the counseling process.

Level I—Internal Listening

The focus here is on *me*. We listen to the other person's words and consider them only as they relate to us. For example, the listener may be deciding how to respond before hearing what the other person has to say. Internal listening is egotistical and involves a great deal of distracting and judgmental thoughts. Our clients and their families may engage only in level I listening; our job is to move everyone up into levels II and III.

Level II—Focused Listening

At this level, the listener gives complete attention to the speaker's words and their meaning. Deep focused listening is like a meditative process and requires full concentration. When we meditate, we focus intently on our breath, whereas when we listen at level II, we focus on the client's words. This is the pathway to becoming fully present. In addition, as level II listeners, we function as a mirror reflecting back the client's words so that he can hear himself. As summarized by Miller and Katz (2014):

> In listening as an ally, we listen deeply and with full attention, viewing others as partners on the same side of the table. We look for value in the speaker's perspectives and build on what they say. We engage with others in the conviction that we are all in this together. We open the door for collaboration to take place and for breakthroughs to arise.

Level III—Global Listening

At level III, we listen with all of our senses, maintaining awareness of the client's eye contact, facial expressions, vocal intonations, body language, posture, mood, and energy. As successful Global Listeners, we fully engage our emotional intelligence and intuition. For example, we pay attention to our clinical intuition and verbalize those hunches according to the client's mood, stage in the process, readiness, and temperament; we do this with sensitivity and tact. One valuable tool for tuning into our intuition is meditation (see Chapter 2).

Ask Yourself

1. Provide a personal example of each level of listening.
   - Level I (Internal Listening)

- Level II (Focused Listening)

- Level III (Global Listening)

2. Write about how the different levels of listening may apply to any supervisor–trainee relationship.

3. Assume roles with a partner: One is the listener, and the other will be the speaker. The listener must listen to the speaker at level I Listening. Level I means that the listener has his own agenda, interrupts, hijacks the agenda, fades in his listening, and uses negative facial expressions and body language.

   Now, switch roles and repeat the exercise.

   Write how you felt as you played each role. Compare how you felt speaking and listening at level I as opposed to Level II. (At first this exercise may feel awkward for both parties, however, with practice, level II listening will become comfortable, even natural.)

4. Select one specific listening behavior that you realize is a problem (a roadblock such as interrupting). Attempt to control this behavior for an hour during the weekend. Build on each success. Discuss in class.

In a helping profession, we may want to fix those who share their thoughts and feelings with us. Often, however, our efforts may be less effective than just listening would be. By genuinely focusing on hearing the client's or family's feelings, reflecting back and paraphrasing what we hear in our own words, we allow them to process their emotions and allow them to come to their own conclusions. When we listen deeply, follow the client's lead, and reflect back, we receive clues to form a relevant and productive response (Andrews, 2004).

LISTENING ROADBLOCKS

The following behaviors interfere with empathic and effective listening. As you read through the roadblocks, notice which ones apply to you.

Mind Chatter

Whom are you listening to when someone speaks? When we ask our students this question, they usually say that they are listening to the speaker. In fact, they're more likely giving their attention to their own *mind chatter*. Mind chatter comes from our inner voices, which stem from both internal interferences, such as hunger, thirst, boredom, thoughts, and judgments, and external environmental interferences, such as background noise and other conversations. When mind chatter grips our attention, we are not fully present to the speaker.

True empathic listening requires us to consistently lower the volume of our inner mind chatter. We sometimes recommend visualizing turning down a dial in our minds. We must also train ourselves to make our minds blank, rendering our interactions all about the client. The students and clinicians may need to "make their minds blank" by learning how to visualize "bundling" or compartmentalizing their interfering thoughts, so that they create a clear mind for deep listening (Craig & Hess, 2010).

Hijacking the Agenda

> *Most people do not listen with the intent to understand; they listen with the intent to reply.*
>
> Stephen Covey, 1989

Listening at levels II and III demands that we resist shifting the focus of the conversation to ourselves, also known as *hijacking the agenda* (Whitworth, 2007). Some of us must break the habit of interrupting. We must recognize how often we change the topic or direction of the conversation without warning or agreement.

Already Always Listening

Sometimes we think we are listening, yet we are actually making assumptions. We'll react to the speaker as if we already know just what he's going to say (after all, we already heard his future words in our minds). When we are *already always listening* (Bry & Erhard, 1977), we interfere with the flow of communication. This phrase also refers to the fact that we often perceive people based on how they've been or how we've perceived them to be in the past. We may identify those who we are already always listening to because they constantly repeat their complaints about life and rarely acknowledge the positive. They may interrupt, dominate conversations, talk incessantly, rarely stay on topic, and fervently impose their opinions. This is a form of level I listening and is ego based.

Given the history of those we are already always listening to and our assumptions, we respond to them out of this knowledge. On the other hand, we may then be surprised if the other person's behavior does not manifest in the way we anticipated. It may be difficult to see that individual from an alternative perspective because we were viewing them as they have always been in the past.

Just as we make assumptions about others, so do others maintain reasons to anticipate our words and behaviors. When we are already always listeners, we're cheating ourselves, and one another, of the chance to grow. The key to escaping this feedback loop is self-awareness.

Ask Yourself

Describe already always listening as it pertains to your listening or how others listen to you.

Emotional Triggers

When another person's words stir our insecurities, we may feel emotionally triggered and go on the defensive. Then whatever the speaker says becomes all about us; we are listening through a narrow perspective and are no longer fully present in our listening. This may occur when a supervisor is giving feedback to a student-clinician, when a clinician is counseling a parent, or when a parent is commenting to a teenager. We may then seek out people who will agree with and validate our upset and perspective.

If we choose to surround ourselves with people who agree with and validate us all the time, we may think we have good relationships. In fact, these relationships maintain our belief that we're right and the other person is wrong. In some cases, if we complain to a group of friends about something or someone, and each person validates our upset, our complaint becomes stronger. For example, we have witnessed students complaining in groups about instructors, clinical supervisors, the administration, and the workload. The complaint seems to gather strength and everyone is in agreement. It is rare for a student to listen to a differing perspective or to have the courage to give one.

Emotional triggers occur in many situations and settings. We therefore need to be aware of how our defensive postures shut down our listening in a communicative exchange. For example, if a clinician hears a parent's comments as a criticism of his work, he may fall into a defensive posture. This, in turn, affects the clinician's communication with the parents, which may have an impact on the relationship. Sometimes a clinician may hear parents' words as critical and unsympathetic to their child's struggle, rather than empathizing with the parents' struggle. This too may distort the clinician's listening and affect communication. We must self-manage these reactions by developing awareness and understanding of our reactions, evaluating where these reactions may stem from, and how we hear and interpret the message.

Ask Yourself

When have you become defensive, shut down, and stopped listening? Describe a personal, academic, and/or professional experience.

Multitasking

Another roadblock is multitasking. M. Scott Peck, MD, PhD (1978) clearly describes that it is impossible to listen deeply and do something else at the same time. Many people today believe they can do both simultaneously. This type of multitasking precludes deep focused listening. Under these circumstances we are not fully present to the people in front of us or their words. We lose out on fully understanding the other person's message. As a result, we may not get to know the other individual as well as we may have if we would have deeply listened. When we listen fully, we demonstrate to the other that we value and respect him. For our children, deep listening demonstrates our love.

Ask Yourself

1. Recall a time when you or another responded to a text or phone call during dinner table conversation. How did this impact your listening?

2. As a parent, have you ever had your child attempt to speak to you while you were already engaged in another activity?

Many parents have noted how frustrating this can be since it is nearly impossible to listen deeply while doing something else. This situation is particularly difficult for children who stutter, who require the parent's full attention when speaking.

Occasionally a parent brings several children to a therapy session with me (BTA). While one child is in session, the others will play in the waiting room. When the session is over, everyone enters and there is the usual activity and rivalry that occurs between siblings. Sometimes there is a screaming baby. Parents often request to have a deeper one-on-one conversation with me. When I comment about the distractions, they usually respond that they can handle it. I acknowledge that it may be so, for them; however, it would be difficult for me to provide the level of listening that is demanded for this type of exchange. We then set up a convenient time for the two of us to speak free of interruptions.

OVERCOMING ROADBLOCKS

The roadblocks we have presented (mind chatter, hijacking the agenda, emotional triggers, multitasking, defensiveness, and resistance), keep us stuck in inauthentic and ineffective listening. To serve as models for the students, clients, and families we work with, we must overcome our own resistance and know our own stumbling blocks. The following suggestions may help us deepen our authentic listening.

Taking Personal Responsibility in Listening

When we take personal responsibility for our listening, it means that we are willing to turn down the volume of our mind chatter and notice the influence of our filters. We acknowledge that we must learn to recognize the assumptions we make, and realize that we do not always know people's reasons for the things they do or say. We suggest trying the following:

- Instead of rushing to conclusions, we could ask curious and open questions, free of defensiveness.

- Instead of hijacking the agenda, we could wait for our turn to speak and avoid intruding or overreacting.

- If we must interrupt a conversation, we could alert the speaker. For example, we might say, "I need to interrupt for a moment."

- If we need clarification from the speaker, we could ask a question, such as, "Do you mean _____?" or "Would you please clarify _____?"

- To determine whether we have heard the client correctly, we might check in (Whitworth, 2007) periodically by asking him a question such as, "Is _____ what you are saying?"

- If we require repetition because our mind has wandered, we admit it by saying, "I'm sorry, I may have lost my focus for a second. Would you please repeat what you just said?"

- As with all challenges, people need to make a choice in the moment between listening and multitasking. Two examples of taking personal responsibility for listening are in Boxes 5-3 and 5-4.

BOX 5-3

An example of taking personal responsibility comes from an anecdote about my mother (BTA). My mother enjoys talking, and once she moved from New York to Florida, she depended on telephone contact to keep in touch with me. When I called her, I felt as if she talked continuously, and there was no opportunity to interject a word. As soon as she picked up the phone, my mother would relay every detail of every day since we'd last spoken.

(continued)

Box 5-3 (continued)

Since our "conversations" fell into this pattern consistently, I would move into a place of already always listening, assuming that this tendency would repeat itself—and it did. Finally, after many months of frustration, I realized that I needed to assume responsibility for my listening as well as for my speaking. I decided to communicate my feelings with sensitivity and love. I asked my mom if I could have a turn to share something with her.

She welcomed the opportunity. I explained that even though I loved to hear about her, sometimes I would love to tell her about my own children and grandchildren. My mother's response was thrilling. "Of course, darling," she said. "Please let me know the minute we get on the phone that you have something to say. I do realize that I go on and on." My mother turned 92 years old in November 2015, and I am very fortunate to communicate with her in such an authentic way. I learned to let go of already always listening because it was keeping me stuck, and instead I took personal responsibility for my communication.

Box 5-4

A coaching client of mine (CSR) often calls between sessions. When she does, I always give her a heads-up about how much time she will have for the phone call. During one conversation, the client expressed her appreciation that I set these parameters at the outset. The client noted that my behavior demonstrated both self-respect and respect for her. The client further relayed that she now uses this approach with family members who constantly call her and detain her for extended periods of time. Being up front about her boundaries has opened up the opportunity for her to be more present to listen to others. Taking personal responsibility for her listening gave my client a feeling of control and raised her self-esteem.

Although it may feel uncomfortable to ask for clarification or repetition when our mind has wandered, it shows respect for the speaker and is important for our comprehension. It also demonstrates that we value the speaker's message. As with all challenges, people need to make a choice in the moment between listening and multitasking.

Some individuals are more impulsive and lack the self-control to listen fully. The good news is, as we have discussed, focused listening can be taught and learned. This work is particularly important in the clinical realm.

We suggest that each family member provides 5 minutes of one-on-one shared time, on a set schedule, with the child who is in therapy. In this way, the child experiences focused listening and turn-taking on a regular basis. We also suggest that family members raise their hands at the dinner table for a turn to talk. In this way, everyone is listening and all children are heard.

Ask Yourself

1. Write about a time when you did not take personal responsibility for your listening, specific to the following:

   a. In an everyday situation

   b. In a clinical situation

Silence and the Creative Pause

Another way to overcome the roadblocks of mind chatter, hijacking the agenda, emotional triggers, multitasking, and defensiveness is in the use of silence. The use of silence is an important and undervalued aspect of listening in our culture. We often avoid silence out of the fear of losing our audience, appearing uninformed, or feeling awkward. Sometimes we speak just to fill our perception of a void. On the other hand, many Native American and Eastern cultures value silence as a form of centering, focusing, reflecting, and respect for elders. These cultures associate silence with wisdom and power (Klopf, 1998; Yum, 1987).

Rather than fearing silence, we can learn to value it. By allowing for a pause during an interaction, we are signaling the other person to speak, allowing him to begin without interrupting. Silence and pausing in conversational turn-taking and listening play an essential role in effective communication.

A *creative pause* is a break in the conversational interaction that may have a powerful impact. For example, when used effectively, the silence may allow an individual to process information, access his feelings, organize his thoughts, and enhance the meaning of his words. During assessment and treatment, we have found that, if we trust in this process, the client will fill the space.

Ask Yourself

How does silence affect your social and clinical interactions? Write an example of each.

PARENTS, CHILDREN, AND LISTENING

In a counseling situation, we must attend to the parents' ability to listen. In many cases, parents are able to listen for the first few minutes at the conclusion of a diagnostic session; however, as soon as they hear stressful news, they figuratively leave the room or shut down. Luterman (2008) asserted that clinicians must avoid spouting technical information to a parent when first discussing a child's difficulties. It is best, he suggested, to encourage parents to ask questions and then answer them clearly and directly without overwhelming them with long explanations.

We have found that sometimes the parent will need more than the 5 minutes at the end of a therapy session to process his child's progress. In these cases, we suggest setting up a phone conference or a separate meeting, so that both the clinician and family member will be available to concentrate and listen. When explained honestly and clearly, parents will appreciate the clinician's effort to fully focus on their child's struggle and on their questions.

Often grandparents are involved in a child's therapy. This family dynamic is common in various cultures or in multigenerational homes. It is most important for the clinician to understand this, so that the grandparents' influence is clear. Many parents may be caught between listening to the recommendations of the clinician and the possible differing opinions heard from their own parents, other family members, and friends. It is the role of the clinician, when listening to the confusion parents express, to help them sort out the ideas. As we listen, reflect on their confusion, and clarify the goals, we are building a working partnership for the benefit of their child. Our ability to listen empathically and nonjudgmentally will foster a strong connection among parent, clinician, and child.

Children also need to learn about listening. In our practices, we work on listening skills at the level that the children are able to handle. We wait our turn and discuss choices and options (Faber & Mazlish, 2012; Ginott, 1969). We have had older clients fill out listening surveys to become aware of these listening strengths and weaknesses. Discussions about listening have affected the work we do with persons who stutter, so that the focus is not only on their speech fluency but also on their ability to listen deeply to others. It is also essential, as clinicians and instructors, for us to be strong listening models for our students, clinicians, clients, and the families we work with and counsel.

Ask Yourself

Answer the following questions to apply the information presented in this chapter. Address these subjects personally, academically, and/or professionally.

1. What have you learned about yourself and others as listeners? Include observations about the tendency to do the following:

   ○ Interrupt

- Take over the conversation

- Change direction of a conversation without agreement and warning

- Not waiting for the pause which invites a response

- Ignore what someone has just said

- Change another's intent to your own

- Try to control a reaction

- Become defensive instead of listening

- Try to fix rather than to listen to what someone is requesting, saying, expressing, and feeling

2. Are you beginning to ask for clarification or repetition to better understand what another person is saying? See the following comments and questions to help articulate your need for clarification:
   ○ "Let me see if I understand what you are saying…"
   ○ "Do you mean…"
   ○ "I'm not sure if I'm following your line of thinking …"

3. In what other ways are you taking responsibility for your listening?

4. How are you dealing with silence and pausing? Do they make you uncomfortable or do you view them as opportunities to invite a response?

5. What are your listening goals?

KEY CONCEPTS

- Our work as health care professionals is affected by our willingness and ability to listen empathically.
- Most individuals are not aware of the type of listener they are.
- Internal listening (level I) focuses on the *me*.
- Focused listening (level II) focuses on the speaker's words and the meaning behind the words and is a skill that we can improve.
- Global listening (level III) focuses on listening with all the senses and is a skill that we may continue to improve.
- Roadblocks (mind chatter, hijacking the agenda, emotional triggers, multitasking, defensiveness, and resistance) to empathic and effective listening keep us stuck, but, fortunately, can be overcome with practice.

- We are often actually listening to ourselves listen.

- To be a true empathic listener, we must reduce our mind chatter, which stems from internal and external distractions and thoughts.

- Already always listening keeps us stuck because rather than listening, we're anticipating what the speaker is going to say, which may be due to past experience.

- When we listen only from our own experiences and perspectives, we make assumptions and misinterpretations.

- Emotional triggers stem from defensiveness, insecurity, or disagreement with someone else's words and can occur personally, academically, and professionally.

- When we search for agreement and validation about an upset, we tend to fuel the upset.

- Parents' listening may shut down when they are presented with too much information.

- It is essential to take personal responsibility for one's listening by requesting repetition, clarification, or setting boundaries on timing and/or time allotted.

- Silence and the creative pause allow everyone to process information, access feelings, and organize thoughts.

- We must learn from and be sensitive to other cultures about the value of silence and about the role that transgenerational factors play in decision making for our clients.

- Altering weak listening habits may be difficult; this requires consistent awareness and practice.

- How we listen affects how we speak and how we speak affects how we listen.

REFERENCES

Andrews, M. A. (2004). Clinical issues: Counseling techniques for speech-language pathologists. *SIG 1 Perspectives on Language, Learning, and Education, 11*(1), 3–8.

Bry, A., & Erhard, W. (1977). *EST: 60 hours that transform your life.* New York, NY: Avon Books.

Covey, S. (1989). *The 7 habits of highly effective people.* New York, NY: Simon & Schuster.

Craig, W., & Hess, R. (2010). *Coach training alliance learning accelerator* [CD]. Boulder, CO: Coach Training Alliance.

Faber, A., & Mazlish, E. (2012). *How to talk so kids will listen & listen so kids will talk.* New York, NY: Simon & Schuster.

Ginott, H. (1969). *Between parent and child: New solutions to old problems.* New York, NY: Avon Books.

Kimsey-House, H., Kimsey-House, K., Sandahl, P., & Whitworth, L. (2011). *Co-active coaching: Changing business, transforming lives.* Boston, MA: Nicholas Brealey Publishing.

Klopf, D. W. (1998). *Intercultural encounters: The fundamentals of intercultural communication.* Englewood, CO: Morton.

Luterman, D. (2008). *Counseling persons with communication disorders and their families* (5th ed.). Austin, TX: Pro-Ed.

Maggiani, R. (2009.) How to truly listen. *Solari.* Retrieved from www.solari.net/toward-humanity/2009/09/29/how-to-truly-listen

Miller, F. A., & Katz, J. H. (2014). 4 keys to accelerating collaboration. *OD PRACTITIONER, 46*(1), 6-11.

Ouellette, S. E. (2004). Clinical issues: Applications of solution-focused concepts to the practice of speech-language pathology. *SIG 1 Perspectives on Language, Learning, and Education, 11*(1), 8–14.

Peck, M. S. (1978). *The road less travelled: A new psychology of love, traditional values and spiritual growth.* New York, NY: Touchstone.

Shafir, R. Z. (2003). *The Zen of listening: Mindful communication in the age of distraction.* Wheaton, IL: Quest Books.

Whitworth, L. (2007). *Co-active coaching: New skills for coaching people toward success in work and life.* Mountain View, CA: Davies-Black Publishing.

Yum, J. O. (1987). Korean philosophy and communication. In D. D. Kincaid (Ed.), *Communication theory: Eastern and Western perspectives.* San Diego, CA: Academic Press.

RECOMMENDED WEBSITES

On listening skills. www.skillsyouneed.com/ips/listening-skills.html
On focusing: Human literacy = listening to oneself and listening to another. www.cefocusing.com/coreconcepts/1a2.php

6

Language
The Power of Words

Words have the power to both destroy and heal. When words are both true and kind, they can change the world.

—Andrea Gardner, 2012

LEARNER OUTCOMES

After reading this chapter, the reader will be able to:

1. Discuss personal responsibility in use of language.

2. Identify and describe the word traps highlighted in this chapter.

3. Explain the importance and impact of nonverbal communication.

4. Describe the language of acknowledgment, gratitude, and validation.

A film excerpt on YouTube, *The Power of Words* (Gardner, 2010), opens with a homeless man sitting on the sidewalk of a bustling Manhattan street. On a carton, he's written, "Help me!" It appears that few have stopped to answer his plea. Finally, a woman stops, takes out a pen, and on the man's carton writes, "It's a beautiful day and I can't see it." Immediately, the man begins receiving an outpouring of coins and bills from passersby. When the woman returns, a short while later, the man asks her, "What happened?" She replies, "I just changed the words."

Andrea Gardner, in her book *Change Your Words, Change Your World* (2012) has demonstrated her commitment to teaching others about the impact of their language. As speech-language pathologists and audiologists who counsel clients and their families, we have always been interested in how language affects others and relates to listening. We see this as crucial for our work.

In the late 1980s, I (BTA) had the opportunity to attend the Communication Workshop through Landmark Education. This weekend seminar stressed the importance of the

Stein-Rubin, C., & Adler, B. T. *Counseling in Communication Disorders: Facilitating the Therapeutic Rehabilitation* (pp 85-101).
© 2017 Taylor & Francis Group.

relationship between our listening and speaking and how each influences the other. I was impressed with the wealth of information and began to apply many of the ideas to my personal life as well as to my work at Brooklyn College in New York and in my private practice. I started to search for books on the subject within my field, psychology, and self-help. Although finding specific sources was difficult, the information that follows is a combination of the ideas developed from my readings, seminars, and workshops. Many of the ideas relate to my therapeutic and teaching experiences and the successes that have grown out of the application of this information.

The language we use influences how people listen, what they hear and attend to, and how they will respond. Our language reveals our judgments, attitudes, feelings, personal issues, sensitivity, and the compassion we have for others and for ourselves. In addition, the way we talk to ourselves influences our ensuing feelings, thoughts, and actions. This cycle eventually shapes who we are, both personally and professionally (Helmstetter, 1990). When we pay attention to what we say and monitor and understand the reactions other people have toward us, we may cultivate a synergistic partnership with the client.

In everyday communication, we often speak the words that pop into our heads without giving them much thought. Spontaneous verbal exchange is typical among peers, family members, and colleagues. We tend to think it's natural and normal to interrupt others, to get sidetracked by another's questions or by our own wandering thoughts, and to steer a conversation away from its point. Some believe that as long as a continuous verbal exchange is happening, so is effective communication.

Some student-clinicians admit that they rarely complete their conversations; they insist that interruptions and topic changes are what make a conversation unfold naturally. These same students have insisted in their early training that it is not necessary to fully listen to each other in a social situation. This attitude comes from the belief that interruptions are typical and do not interfere with the ability to listen. We question this point with our students because we have learned that success in our field requires us to practice focused listening and to carefully choose our words. If one does not make the decision to become conscientious about one's speaking, and practice this conscientiousness often, how could one expect to be successful when engaging with clients? As our students learn more about listening and speaking in our courses, they learn to emphasize and apply the principles of listening, along with word choices and the importance of topic maintenance. The student-clinicians have expressed that working on these skills has had a notable impact on their communication socially, academically, and professionally.

UNEXPECTED REACTIONS IN A CONVERSATION

Sometimes in conversation, we get a totally unexpected response and wonder what happened. Our tendency might be to amend our words without sufficient thought. Sometimes this hasty repair may provoke a greater communication breakdown. We may find ourselves floundering and lost without knowing how to get back on track in the discussion. Box 6-1 provides an example of an unexpected response.

Box 6-1

Bill and Sam were meeting for lunch. Sam was worried about his imminent back surgery, and he mentioned to Bill that he would undergo this procedure the next week. Concerned about his friend, Bill replied, "You know, there have been many back surgeries that have been useless and have even caused harm." Suddenly livid, Sam stood up from the table and shouted, "You are my good friend; how dare you say something like that to me!" Bill, shocked and perplexed, tried to glean what he had said that had upset Sam so much. Although Bill tried to make his point a different way, Sam seemed to become angrier and more upset.

Although Bill meant well, he was not being fully empathetic. Had he listened deeply, he would have realized that Sam was not seeking advice and that Sam had already committed to having the surgery. Bill would have also realized that Sam's overreaction stemmed from his fear about the surgery. Sam obviously needed support, encouragement, and, most of all, someone who listened deeply and chose his words carefully. Had Bill done these things, he would have experienced a very different result. Box 6-2 offers another example of the importance of choosing our words carefully.

Box 6-2

Mary went to her cardiologist for a follow-up visit regarding her fluctuating blood pressure. After the examination, the doctor said that she was disappointed with the results considering that Mary has been on medication and had just come from a Pilates class. The discussion that followed, between physician and patient, caused increasing anxiety for Mary. Had the doctor used more positive and encouraging language, she could have gotten her message across and diminished Mary's growing anxiety. For example, the doctor could have said, "Mary, your blood pressure is improving. Let's continue our work to lower it further." Mary would have then left the office encouraged and strengthened, feeling that she was on the right path, rather than disappointed.

Once words are spoken, it is difficult to retract them. This patient–doctor interaction in Box 6-2 left the patient experiencing anxiety over her blood pressure for a considerable length of time. If the doctor had chosen her words more carefully, the patient might have had a greater sense of well-being and confidence in the process.

These *communication breakdowns* (Owens, 2011) or miscommunications require our awareness, attention, and sensitivity. Although we are not responsible for another person's listening, we are responsible for the language we use, our choice of words, and the intention behind whatever it is we have to say. We are, of course, also responsible for our own listening.

Nonverbal Communication

The mark of success in spoken communication is that the listener receives the message that the speaker intends to convey. A client's understanding of a clinician's intended message is dependent on the clinician's words and nonverbal cues. According to Small (2012), 65% of conversation is nonverbal. In other words, the individual's body language may be more telling than her words about the way she really feels.

Our *body language* (posture, stance, head position, facial expressions, and gestures) sends significant nonverbal cues. The *suprasegmental aspects* of our communication (intonation, timing, stress, loudness, and rate of speech) provide the color and melody to our words and strengthens our message. All of these aspects of speech give the listener insight into the speaker and what the speaker is feeling. If there is a discrepancy between the nonverbal and verbal aspects of the speaker's message, oftentimes the nonverbal is more telling.

Similarly, Andrews (2004) discusses the *intent of the message*, as opposed to strictly the content, as giving the message its meaning. For example, when a clinician asks a parent a question, such as, "Can you tell me what you do when you play with Alice?" the question needs to come from a place of neutrality and a nonjudgmental stance. If the tone and body posture reveal judgment, the parent may become defensive. Therefore, the question must come from a genuinely curious and supportive place. The intention of the clinician must be to acknowledge the parent for playing appropriately with her child. This attitude paves the way for a more positive parental reaction to be more available to the learning process (Box 6-3).

Box 6-3

A parent of a 2-year-old child called my (BTA) office with concerns about her son Danny's speech and language. She described him as very energetic and unable to sit still and play interactively. The mother explained that her son lost focus whenever she engaged in an activity with him. She requested an evaluation as soon as possible. After listening to her description, I asked her if she would be willing to bring a toy they play with together at home so that I could observe them interacting. She agreed.

During the diagnostic session, I asked them to play on the floor together while I sat in a corner. As Danny demonstrated that he could build with his mom, she immediately shrieked loudly with joy and clapped her hands enthusiastically—the sound was piercing. Danny instantly jumped up and began running around the room out of control. Mom sadly expressed that this is what happens at home.

As soon as he calmed down, I suggested that they do this again and that this time she use a quieter tone and endearingly praise her son without the hand clapping. She did, and they played beautifully together for several minutes without interruption. Mom was stunned and said she always thought that praising had to be exaggerated with children. I reinforced her desire to praise her son and suggested that he probably needed a more gentle and quieter approach. I told her that she did quite well, and we were then able to move forward with the evaluation.

This little boy was sensitive to noise and vocal tone. As soon as his mother was made aware of this, she altered the way that she interacted with her child. Danny's mom shared the events with family members so that everyone was aware of the best ways to work and play with him.

A client may express excitement through the emotion in her tone or through the content of her message. The clinician may then glean the real meaning of her statement. For example, a client who stutters may say she has been using her new way of talking and has been fluent. As she continues to talk about her speaking, she comments that she probably doesn't sound as natural as other people. The clinician may pick up cues from her voice and the content of the message. In this case, it is important for the clinician to probe the client about how she hears herself as different from other people (Riley, 2002).

It is also important to pay attention to eye contact, body posture, and gestures. For example, if an individual's arms are open, she may be conveying receptivity, whereas tightly folded arms may reflect protectiveness or rigid ideas. When the speaker clenches her fist, fidgets, or rubs her hands together continuously, it may imply nervousness and anxiety. By observing facial expressions, the listener may also pick up on the speaker's interest level, sincerity, concern, and compassion. For example, when a client clenches her jaw, she may be feeling anxiety.

Both the speaker and listener shift back and forth, changing roles while attending to the nonverbal cues, suprasegmentals, words, and intention behind the message. This continuous cycle is referred to as the *communication chain* (Denes & Pinson, 1993). Because there is always a connection between listening and speaking, it is the feedback that alerts us to the success of the interaction.

Ask Yourself

Think about the following and write a brief response to each:

1. Do you believe the language you use empowers the other person and opens up possibility?

2. Do your words lead to collaboration with your clients?

3. Do your words lead to collaboration with your friends and/or family members?

4. Which nonverbal cues have encouraged your participation in a conversation? Which have closed you down?

PERSONAL RESPONSIBILITY IN LANGUAGE

If one of our goals is to trust in our clients' and family members' wisdom and to view them as experts on their own lives, then the intention behind the message, the language we use, and our nonverbal communication, are the vehicles for conveying this trust. Taking *personal responsibility* for our speaking is as important as it is for listening (see the section "Taking Personal Responsibility in Listening" in Chapter 5). We must be cognizant of the words we use so that they empower our clients rather than provoke their defensive postures. How we choose to listen and how we choose to speak must work together without the interference of negative interpretations and assumptions. As Bry and Erhard (1977) said, "Speak without offending, and listen without defending."

For us to assume personal responsibility for our speaking, the following points are important:

- We must be self-aware and lose our need to be right.
- We must be willing to admit to interrupting the client.
- We must not make assumptions about what the client has said.
- We must choose our own words thoughtfully.
- We must ask our clients and/or family members for clarification when needed, such as, "Are you referring to your father or your stepfather?"
- If a client misinterprets or misunderstands our words, it is our responsibility to clarify and rephrase to the best of our ability.
- Use specific language and avoid technical terminology, unless requested.

Family members or clients may ask the same questions a number of times. Student-clinicians may lose patience in these situations. The truth is, if one takes the family member's perspective, she may understand what is behind the repeated question. The client or family member may be letting the clinician know she still does not understand, something may be missing in the explanation, or that she may need more reassurance. This is a frequent occurrence in treatment. It is also beneficial to check in with the client to ascertain that she understood the information that was delivered (Kimsey-House, Kimsey-House, Sandahl, & Whitworth, 2011).

We often think that clarification is about simply repeating ourselves. We hope that if we do, we will get the response we want. Most often, repeating words in the same way clarifies nothing. We suggest repeating yourself for clarification purposes no more than twice (say it once and repeat it only once more). If the other person does not respond to what we meant to convey, there is clearly a communication breakdown. We are then responsible for figuring out what went wrong, what the other person understood, and what remains unclear.

When we honor each other by offering clarification as well as openly receiving requests for clarification, we have created an opportunity to change the language, so that the message is received as intended. We aim to teach student clinicians how to catch themselves, to be self-aware sooner rather than later, and not to sweep the problem under the rug.

Asking Permission

Another way we may take personal responsibility for our speaking is by asking permission to make suggestions, for example, "May I offer a suggestion?" By doing this, we empower the client or family member in the relationship and demonstrate that we understand the limits and boundaries of the relationship. In turn, we foster mutual respect and the development of a partnership paradigm (Kimsey-House et al., 2011).

Ask Yourself

Write about a situation in which you might apply each of the following phrases and questions:

- "May I offer a suggestion?"

- "Are you willing to consider another possibility?"

- "May I offer you some feedback on that?"

- "Let me clarify what I meant."

- "I would like to explain this in a different way."

- "Do you want to ask me additional questions so that we are on the same page?"

- "Is there anything I said that was not clear? Please feel free to ask me questions."

WORD TRAPS

We frequently choose the wrong words because we're on autopilot or because we are not aware of the impact the words will have on another person. We're surprised when we do not get the response we were hoping to receive, unaware that our language shut down the communication. Let's explore some of the *word traps* we use when talking to children, as well as adults. Likewise, we also react when someone uses these words when speaking to us.

Should Versus Could

Louise Hay (1984) has spent years working with individuals with catastrophic illnesses who are dealing with the guilt and resentment of *should*. She talks about the burden of *should* and how it eliminates choices. It's the no-possibility way of thinking, the dead end. *Should guilt* eventually leads to anger because it makes a person feel dictated to and stuck. When we speak to our clients and families, we must remove the pressure of *should* and provide the freedom of *could*.

Notice your reaction when you hear or use the word *should*. Should precludes options and shuts down the creative thinking that we need to help us generate other perspectives and solutions. It creates a sense of pressure by provoking feelings of obligation and force. Some common, often internal, responses to *should* include, "No I don't have to," or "I don't feel like it," or "I can't," and "Who said so?" In other words, we react to *should* with resistance. We get stuck and feel guilty that we are disappointing others and ourselves. Then we may become angry, resentful, and defensive about why we have not completed or accomplished anything. In both our thinking and our speaking, if we change *should* to *could*, we open up opportunities (Hay, 1984).

We have adapted Louise Hay's ideas on language in our clinical practice. When a therapist tells a parent, "You *should* do this every day," the parent thinks, "Yes, there are many things I *should* do and just can't." Then the parent may feel guilty about not meeting the goal. When that guilt, subsequent anger, and resentment build, it's not uncommon for parents and clients to quit therapy. Then everyone feels like a failure, and the healing process has reached a dead end. Instead, try asking the parent what she could do, "How often could you practice?" By asking her to honestly assess what is possible in his busy everyday life, the parent may gain control over the situation. The *locus of control* (source of control) has become internal rather than external (Manning, 2009).

Together, create a plan that makes sense for all parties involved. This is the way we are able to assist parents to be part of the process, to have some control over the decisions, and to feel respected and understood. When empowered in this way, the parent and/or child are more likely to take ownership and follow through with practice. When we change the way we express our message to the parents, the results may be profound. We respond more positively when we have choices; we experience less pressure and guilt. The word *could* allows one to choose what to do, how to do it, and if she even wants to do it at all.

Ask Yourself

1. Notice your *should* vs *could* language. Make a list of 10 *should* statements for yourself. Sit with the list and tune in to your feelings and reactions. Now cross out *should* and write *could*. How does it feel? Do you respond better to pressure or to choice?

1.	6.
2.	7.
3.	8.
4.	9.
5.	10.

2. How do you feel when someone uses the word *should* in conversation with you?

3. Write a few *should* statements for your client's parents. How might the parent react? Try to change the language to allow for choice.

And and But Language

Remember a time when someone praised you for your efforts on a job or on your appearance, only to follow the compliment up with a *but*. What impact did the compliment have on you? Did it validate or deflate you? *But* is one of the most commonly used words in our vocabulary. We must remain mindful of our *but* language. Generally, when people hear, "You look great, but _____" or "The lesson was well done, but you didn't do _____," they do not experience the compliment that came before that little word, only whatever came after it—the critical part. When using the word *but*, the negative part of the feedback tends to overshadow the positive, and the positive part is excluded.

On the other hand, *and* is inclusive. When we change *but* to *and*, we change the message we're sending and open the lines of communication. *And* lets us expand on things we say without provoking distance, disappointment, or negativity. When speaking as a clinician, supervisor, or instructor, attempt to limit the use of *but* from your feedback to experience more effective communication.

Try incorporating the phrase *Yes and* into your vocabulary rather than *Yes but* _____. Consider the difference between, "You did a really nice job, *but* you didn't _____," vs "You did a really nice job *and* next time you may want to add _____." The latter won't provoke feelings of failure and inadequacy in the listener, so she'll be able to hear your suggestions better. We're not saying you must cut *but* from your vocabulary; rather, use it sparingly and only after you've thought about how it will sound to your listener.

Ask Yourself

1. Think about your *but* vs *and* language. Consider it from the point of view of both the speaker and the listener. Rewrite the following statements with *and* instead of *but*. What is your reaction?

   ○ I want to visit my mother but she annoys me.

○ I try to listen to my supervisor but what she says angers me.

○ I should do what my boss says but I disagree with him.

The Impact of Can't

Similar to the preceding word traps, the word *can't* is limiting in communication. It can be provocative, reflect a personal fear of failure, or indicate resistance to change. Replacing can't with more positive language will allow you to deliver your messages in the most encouraging and supportive ways possible.

Provocative Can't

Whether in a clinical setting, at school, or at home, when we tell a child, "You can't," we're holding up a red flag. We're not talking about our instinctive use of the command when a child is in immediate danger, but rather about less charged situations, such as "You can't have dessert now," "You can't go outside at this moment," "You can't watch more television," or "You can't play a game until your work's done."

When adults tell children they "can't," a power struggle often ensues. When we point out this dynamic to a parent during a counseling session, she'll readily acknowledge that in the wake of "You can't," her child becomes increasingly difficult.

Parents and children aren't the only ones who get caught in the can't power struggle. The language is just as charged for teachers and students, therapists and clients, and supervisors and student-clinicians. For better results, try exchanging *can't* for words that create options. For example, if a child says, "I want dessert now," instead of saying, "You can't," try, "Do we have dessert before or after dinner?" (Shure & DiGeronimo, 1996). Then follow up by offering her a choice of dessert.

In a therapy situation try, "Since you are in charge today, you get to decide which activity to do first. Do you want to use the computer, read a storybook, or play a board game?" If you let the other person come up with her own way to solve a situation, she'll feel more empowered and less inclined to fight. For more suggestions, specifically for children, we recommend books by Drs. Faber, Mazlish, and Shure.

What happens when you suggest to your adult client who stutters that she openly disclose that she is someone who stutters? She is initially surprised and resistant to this suggestion and will often respond, "I can't." Try coaching your client with questions such as, "Who do you feel is the most comfortable person for you to share with about your stuttering?" This shift away from "I can't" may need to be accomplished in small incremental steps. If you allow the other person, child or adult, to come up with a realistic way to resolve her situation, she will be more empowered, and will be less inclined to argue.

Fear of Failure Can't

When a parent or teacher hears a child say, "I can't do that," the reaction is usually, "Yes you can!" This kind of exchange may also lead to a power struggle, each person insisting on her own point of view, until everyone is frustrated and nothing has been resolved.

Next time an individual says, "I can't," think about what lies beneath that word—laziness, stubbornness, fear, or something else? Rather than contradict the person, it's up to us to encourage and support her. For example, we might ask, "What about this is difficult for you?" or "What part of this do you know how to do?" We might suggest, "Show me what you can do," or "Let me show you how to do it."

If you are a supervisor, acknowledge that your student has fears and concerns about meeting her responsibilities. She might think "I can't" because she doesn't know how to carry out a suggestion. We need to empathize and provide support by modeling and explaining what to do. Recall how, as a new supervisor, you might have experienced similar concerns; for example, perhaps you thought, "I don't know enough to tell this person what to do" (Box 6-4).

Box 6-4

When my (BTA) son graduated from high school, we took a family trip to Bermuda. We decided that each of us would select an activity in which all of us would participate. I selected horseback riding, and everyone agreed. When both of my children selected snorkeling, I froze and said, "I can't do it; I don't swim well and I am afraid of the water." They refused to let me off the hook. In a panic, I called the snorkeling company and asked if I could come on board for the ride and not snorkel. They agreed to my plan. I put my plan into place without arguing with my children. Everyone suited up and immediately jumped into the water; I sat there taking my time. The instructor returned and asked me to hurry. I explained that I was not planning to snorkel and proceeded to explain, "I can't do this, I have a fear of the water." He said, "Okay, why don't you get the equipment and sit near the edge of the boat?" My response was simple, "Sure, I can do that." A little while later he returned and said, "Try the mask, hold onto the edge of the boat and just look down." I said, "Sure, I can do that." Of course the scene under the water was breathtaking. Finally, he suggested that I hold onto the edge of the boat and move all around it, making sure to look down and take in the beauty. In the end, he guided our family away from the boat for a full experience.

This was an experience I will never forget. The instructor never pressured, forced, or embarrassed me. Instead, he helped me to handle my fears step by step and reinforced my efforts, thus helping to shift my belief from "I can't" to "I can."

Just as we help our clients by simplifying goals into smaller more manageable steps, or *successive approximation* (Roth & Worthington, 2011), across all speech-language disorders, counseling goals must be broken down this way as well. For example, when we provide carryover goals in counseling, we might initially ask the client to notice the times during her typical day when insecurities and uncertainties reveal themselves (see the section "Inner Critic" in Chapter 9). We would then acknowledge her for successfully completing the task. Secondarily, we might ask the client to journal the way that she reacted to her inner critical voice. Finally, her assignment might be to write down how she managed this critical voice during her daily activities, what the result of this was, and so on.

Resistance to Change Can't

Habits and patterns are often difficult to break. When we are faced with the unfamiliar and asked to do something different, our resistance often kicks in and keeps us stuck. If someone suggests a change—from an instructor asking a student to switch seats to a mother asking her adult child to take over the family business—there may be resistance. Sometimes the resistance remains only in one's mind, and sometimes the person verbalizes it aloud—"I can't." Generally, individuals prefer the status quo, that which is comfortable and familiar. Yet when we allow change to happen, we allow for personal growth.

When we learn to be mindful of our own resistance to change, we have an opportunity to be compassionate for others when they say, "I can't." In this way, we may diffuse a power struggle, overcome fears, and reduce resistance.

Ask Yourself

1. Make a list of five "I can't" statements (e.g., "I can't go to school and work at the same time"). Write about the nature of the limiting language and how to change it to achieve a goal.

2. Write about a time when someone said "can't" to you. How did you feel? How did you react?

3. Write down three things you have said or anticipate saying to a child using the word *can't*. How would you change these statements after reading and practicing this material?

Why

Cognitively and educationally, we teach children to answer *why* questions. By the time children enter elementary school, it is important for them to learn how to infer and understand the motivation of the characters in stories (Owens, 2008). Yet, when it comes to emotionally-based situations, asking "why" can be provocative. For example, the mother of an 11-year-old female client, when reprimanding her daughter, would yell at her asking, "Why are you doing that? What were you thinking?" The child would silently stare into space; she did not explain, excuse herself, or apologize. The child relayed to the clinician that she became frozen from her mother's consistent use of *why*, and the mom became angry about her daughter's lack of remorse.

Another example of the ineffectiveness of *why* is a 7-year-old male client who becomes frustrated with friends or siblings during play. He often hits or pushes the other child as a way of expressing his upset. His mother's response was, "Why did you do that?" She tended to repeat these words over and over, expecting him to explain his action.

The *why* question may sound accusatory, in certain situations, and may often create a defensive reaction. In response to *why*, some children may tend to act out further or shut down and retreat. Furthermore, children often do not clearly understand why they make the choices they do. When asking "why," parents search for the reason behind the child's behavior rather than address the unacceptable behavior. For example, the girl's mother might say, "We do not eat six snacks. Let's choose three of your favorite and save the rest for later." The parent of the young boy may say, "It is not okay to hit and push; let's use our words and practice together." It is important to note that the pitfalls of *why* are as relevant when conversing with adults as they are when talking to children. We suggest that you remain mindful when using this language to foster more open communication.

Ask Yourself

Remember a time you asked a young child why she did something. How did she respond?

The Language of Validation

Validation, in communication counseling, goes one step further than reflective listening. Validating a client's feelings means relating that you understand how she might feel a certain way. When a parent, child, student-clinician, or even a personal friend or family member shares information with us, a frequent response is, "I understand." The use of these words, however, may be provocative in certain contexts. In reality, we do not understand exactly what another person is feeling and experiencing unless we have had the same experience. In a sense, saying, "I understand" may trivialize the experience for the person who is sharing her upset. A student-clinician, or even a seasoned clinician whose life experience is totally different, may not necessarily understand the parent's everyday struggles.

It has been our clinical experience that sometimes the phrase *I understand*, although well intentioned, is not the best choice. These words might be interpreted by a client or family member as meaning, "I understand your experience." On the other hand, if we expand on *I understand* by making it more specific, such as in the sentence, "I understand that you are feeling overwhelmed," *understand* validates the client's emotion rather than her specific struggle.

We suggest saying, "I hear your pain," "I hear the concerns you have," or "Tell me more about the traditions and customs in your family so that I can better understand this situation." These responses encourage the client to share more about what they are feeling. If the client disagrees and corrects the clinician's interpretation of the emotion, accept what they have to say, and discuss it further.

Student-clinicians and new clinicians may be fearful of being wrong when validating a client's emotion. The client will tell you if you are on the right track or off the mark. If the client disagrees with your validation, don't take this personally. The client is merely helping to clarify her emotional experience. Use this information to help to gain a greater understanding of her struggle and to help direct future questions and comments. It is important that the clinician sometimes takes risks and responds effectively to the client's narrative (see Chapters 8 and 9 for elaboration on how to manage negative and limiting beliefs).

Ask Yourself

Has anyone ever responded to you with "I understand," and in your heart you knew that they didn't? Describe.

THE LANGUAGE OF APPRECIATION: ACKNOWLEDGMENT AND GRATITUDE

The deepest principle of human nature is the craving to be appreciated.

—William James

We express our appreciation in terms of *acknowledgment* and *gratitude*. The term *acknowledgment* means "to recognize as being valid or having force or power." Acknowledgment involves being brave enough to step forward and authentically name what you see and feel (Kimsey-House et al., 2011). Acknowledging an individual highlights her internal strengths, thus fostering greater access to those gifts. Ask yourself whether you have acknowledged those individuals who have had the greatest influence on your choices. We often shy away from acknowledging those people who include family members, mentors, colleagues, close friends, acquaintances, and coworkers.

Think about the lost moments when you thought about acknowledging another person and didn't. People are tentative to provide words of acknowledgment. They may feel self-conscious that their words sound cheesy, insincere, or like an attempt to "butter-up" the other individual. They may also worry about making the other person feel uncomfortable about their response. Therefore, delivering acknowledgment is a brave and courageous act. In many ways, acknowledging another individual is more difficult than pointing out what is lacking. When we acknowledge another individual, in many ways, this requires more courage than pointing out what is lacking.

Acknowledging differs from complimenting. A compliment is more superficial, non-specific, and focuses on what the individual did for you rather than on whom they are *being* to you. In contrast, a true acknowledgment is spoken directly to the other person, is specific, is said in the first person, and reflects a tone of admiration. For example:

Compliment: You are a good mother.

Acknowledgment: I see how your child lights up when he sees you—it's apparent that the two of you have a special connection.

In the clinical realm, take a moment and let your client or family member know where she has a unique force or power because acknowledgment is a powerful relationship builder and helps reduce defensiveness. You may want to provide the family with an assignment that instructs them to deliver one acknowledgment per day, verbal or written, to a family member.

In addition, experiment with acknowledgment in everyday life, and pay attention to the impact it can have. When we speak an authentic acknowledgment, the face of the recipient often reveals that she knows it to be true. When we acknowledge ourselves for our accomplishments, strengths, special gifts, dedication, and hard work, it raises our self-confidence, self-esteem, and continued motivation. Notice that acknowledgment can often have a positive physiological effect on mood for both the receiver and giver. Therefore, delivering and receiving appreciation is healthy (Kimsey-House et al., 2011). Imagine attending routine meetings, such as in the workplace or a study group. The protocol at these meetings would be to allot the first 5 minutes for each group member to acknowledge at least one individual in that group for something they admire about her behavior or contribution.

Gratitude is an expression of thanks. Expressions of gratitude, even if ever-so-small, may make the difference in the giver's and receiver's entire day. We frequently postpone expressing our appreciation in this way. Whether it takes the form of a phone call, letter, e-mail, or face-to-face contact (which is the best), we must express our gratitude for the gifts we receive. According to Martin Seligman (2002), studies on gratitude reveal that specific exercises using gratitude, done on a regular basis, are at least as effective in elevating mood as the use of psychiatric medications.

Ask Yourself

1. Notice the effect when you are acknowledged and/or when you take the time to acknowledge a coworker or fellow student. Describe the experience.

2. Martin Seligman (2002) suggested maintaining a gratitude journal on a weekly basis. In the journal, describe three good things that happened each week. Share this information with a partner or read it aloud to yourself. This technique increases our mindfulness on appreciation and has a positive effect on mood.

3. Seligman (2002) also suggested conducting a *gratitude visit*. The purpose of this exercise is to visit an individual who has made a significant impact on your life. Speak your acknowledgment to this person, making sure to maintain eye contact. You may choose to bring a small gift that represents your acknowledgment.

KEY CONCEPTS

- The language we use influences how people listen—what they hear and attend to and how they respond.

- We may think that our natural habits enhance communication, yet they might be both professionally and personally ineffective.

- Although we are not responsible for another's listening, we are responsible for our own speaking—the language we use, our choice of words, and the intention behind whatever we say.

- The language we use and how the listener receives our words can create either a partnership in problem solving or an adversarial situation that precludes growth.

- Body language and the suprasegmental aspects of speech are significant nonverbal cues.

- Taking personal responsibility for our speaking means that we are clear about the intention of our message, consider our word choice in expressing it, use our nonverbal language to support meaning, clarify as needed, and check in to be sure the listener understood the message.

- When we ask permission to make suggestions, we increase the client's power in the relationship.

- When the clinician sets unattainable goals for the parent, the parent is set up for failure, which leads to parental guilt.

- Word traps such as *should*, *but*, and *can't* may provoke parental guilt, preclude options and possibilities, spark negativity, and block effective communication.

- Replace *should* with *could* and *but* with *and* to open up options, encourage possibilities, and ignite positive thinking and reactions.

- *Can't* may be provocative, reflect fear, or provoke resistance to change.

- *Why* language, in an emotional context, can be challenging and provocative.

- The language of validation goes one step beyond reflective listening. Validation means the clinician hears and understands the client's struggles and emotions.

- The words *I understand*, are often simplistic and inauthentic in response to the extent of a client's pain and suffering. These words must be qualified and expanded as follows: "I understand that you feel angry about _____."

- The language of appreciation (acknowledgment and gratitude) is underused and when expressed openly and honestly can build relationships and reduce defensiveness.

REFERENCES

Andrews, M. A. (2004). Clinical issues: Counseling techniques for speech-language pathologists. *SIG 1 Perspectives on Language, Learning, and Education, 11*(1), 3–8.

Bry, A., & Erhard, W. (1977). *EST: 60 hours that transform your life.* New York, NY: Avon Books.

Denes, P. B., & Pinson, E. (1993). *The speech chain: The physics and biology of spoken language.* London, United Kingdom: Macmillan.

Gardner, A. (2010). *The power of words* [Video]. Retrieved from www.youtube.com/watch?v=Hzgzim5m70U

Gardner, A. (2012). *Change your words, change your world.* Carlsbad, CA: Hay House.

Hay, L. L. (1984). *You can heal your life.* Carlsbad, CA: Hay House.

Helmstetter, S. (1990). *What to say when you talk to your self.* New York, NY: Simon & Schuster.

Kimsey-House, H., Kimsey-House, K., Sandahl, P., & Whitworth, L. (2011). *Co-active coaching: Changing business, transforming lives.* Boston, MA: Nicholas Brealey.

Manning, W. H. (2009). *Clinical decision making in fluency disorders* (3rd ed.). San Diego, CA: Singular.

Owens, R. E. (2008). *Language development: An introduction* (7th ed.). New York, NY: Pearson.

Owens, R. E. (2011). *Language development: An introduction* (8th ed.). New York, NY: Pearson.

Riley, J. (2002). Counseling: An approach for speech-language pathologists. *Contemporary Issues in Communication Science and Disorders, 29,* 6–16.

Roth, F. P., & Worthington, C. K. (2011). *Treatment resource manual for speech-language pathologists.* Clifton Park, NY: Delmar Cengage Learning.

Seligman, M. E. (2002). *Authentic happiness: Using the new positive psychology to realize your potential for lasting fulfillment.* New York, NY: Free Press.

Shure, M., & DiGeronimo, T. F. (1996). *Raising a thinking child.* New York, NY: Simon & Schuster.

Small, L. H. (2012). *Fundamentals of phonetics: A practical guide for students* (3rd ed.). New York, NY: Pearson.

7

Developing Strengths

Success means having the courage, the determination, and the will to become the person you believe you were meant to be.

—George A. Sheehan

LEARNER OUTCOMES

After reading this chapter, the reader will be able to:

1. Become familiar with the 24 signature strengths identified by Peterson and Seligman (2004).

2. Identify personal signature strengths.

3. Describe the elements of constructive feedback according to Fredrickson and Dweck.

4. Describe the solution-focused brief therapy (SFBT) model and cite its components.

5. Conduct an SFBT session with another individual.

In 1995, Jack Reimer wrote an article in the *Houston Chronicle* (Holland, 2007) about a particular concert delivered by the great composer and musician, Itzhak Perlman, in Avery Fisher Hall. Facing the reverent silence and eager anticipation of his audience, Perlman rose to begin his performance. The first few bars started out with his usual prowess, and then suddenly, a snap was heard across the otherwise silent concert hall. The snap was the unmistakable sound of a violin string breaking. Without missing a beat, Perlman revised his arrangement to allow for the absence of the fourth string. His performance was even more spectacular than usual, and the audience was astounded, because they realized that he had done his most masterful performance despite the hardship that was thrust upon him.

Each and every one of us has music within us. Martin Seligman and Chris Peterson (2002), pioneers in positive psychology, have described this music as character strengths,

Stein-Rubin, C., & Adler, B. T. *Counseling in Communication Disorders: Facilitating the Therapeutic Rehabilitation* (pp 103-123).

or signature strengths that may be defined as "positive traits reflected in thoughts, feelings, and behaviors. They exist in degrees and can be measured as individual differences." In addition, using our strengths makes us feel invigorated, and when our strengths are involved, activities seem to flow much easier. Seligman and Peterson (2002), through their research, identified the following 24 strengths:

- Curiosity
- Social intelligence
- Leadership
- Citizenship
- Creativity
- Hope
- Persistence
- Spirituality
- Bravery
- Zest
- Prudence
- Modesty/humility
- Self-regulation
- Fairness
- Integrity
- Judgment
- Gratitude
- Kindness
- Love of learning
- Humor
- Love
- Appreciation of beauty
- Perspective/wisdom
- Forgiveness

According to positive psychologists, we all possess all of these strengths to a degree, on a continuum. Some are more prevalent in one person than another, and vice versa. One person's most salient strength might be zest, while another's may be spirituality. The patterns of character strengths that each one of us exhibit are what makes us unique individuals. To determine our patterns of character strengths, we recommend taking the Values in Action (VIA) free survey available at www.viacharacter.org.

Another way to determine signature strengths is to think about a peak experience or a time when you were engaged in something and you absolutely loved the experience. From that experience, Seligman and Peterson (2002) suggest that you search within this experience for strengths and virtues that you notice within yourself. They also suggest asking yourself how your friends might describe you and asking your friends to describe what strengths they notice within you. Students and clients are often surprised at the positive feedback they receive from others about how they come across. The commentary does not seem to fit with their self perception. It is interesting to note that people are generally more focused on their weaknesses and shortcomings than they are on their strengths and virtues.

Ask Yourself

1. Write down three things you like about yourself. You're welcome to ask your friends and family to help you make the list.

2. Another way to discover your dominant strengths is to recall the times when you were at your best and felt strong and successful. Jot down your peak experience(s). Work with a friend if possible. Ask yourself or each other the following questions about each memory:

   ○ What were you doing?

   ○ Why was this experience important to you?

   ○ From this experience, what did you learn about yourself?

   ○ When else in your life have you applied the strengths discovered from your peak experience?

   ○ How successful were you?

3. Write down and compare your strengths from the VIA survey to the ones you discovered from your own experience. Do you see common threads between the attributes you listed and the results of the survey? The combination of all these will provide a clearer picture of your *best self.*

4. Another strengths survey is the Keirsey Temperament Sorter (www.Keirsey.com). Complete this survey online. Click on the box in the upper right-hand corner. You will receive a free detailed printout of your personality profile, one of four archetypes, including highlighted strengths.

The findings and concepts of positive psychology mesh well with our own needs and with the needs of our profession (Holland, 2007). We can apply a strengths-based approach when we deal with a client who is suffering from a life-altering crisis, such as a communication disorder. With that said, one need not be a psychologist to benefit from a strengths perspective. As healers, when a client is faced with a challenge, we must consider our own past experiences and focus on our own strengths to assess how to proceed. By modeling a strengths perspective, we are in a better position to encourage our clients to consider what has worked for them in the past. To tackle the crisis, we can amplify their strengths while also knowing our own. We must do the work to know ourselves before we can help others recognize the work they need to do.

Rather than looking for what's strong, what's working, and what we have accomplished, we often focus on weakness and view ourselves as weak and ineffective. Some of us have been beaten down or rejected; some have shaky self-confidence and give into limiting beliefs; others feel empty as if a part of them is missing. Yet how frequently, despite our limitations, do we rise from the ashes and create something more significant than ever before? For example, what about the Iraq War veteran, missing an arm and a leg, who inspired us by competing and became a finalist on the TV show *Dancing With the Stars*? We've seen children with cancer appear on TV shows, nationwide, to engender hope for people with this illness and for the population at large. We marvel at our clients who, despite their limitations, find their niches and pursue respectable and productive careers.

Let's refer back to the story about Itzhak Perlman, who made lemons out of lemonade. He focused on what was working rather than on what wasn't. He knew his strengths, used these to address his weakness, and showed up bigger and better than ever. Even what we may think of as our imperfections may also turn out to be strengths. Like Itzhak Perlman, we—as clinicians, supervisors, and instructors—must have the capacity to perform in the moment. We must be able to self-manage and have the flexibility and the skills to adapt, adjust, and create out of the challenge. We must know and hone in on our personal and professional strengths and weaknesses. If we maintain a balanced perspective, it helps to foster personal and professional growth (Buckingham & Clifton, 2001; De Shazer, 1988).

Let's examine the following story about how speech-language clinicians lean into strengths to address weaknesses of their clients (Box 7-1).

Box 7-1

One of the clients I (CSR) supervised presented with aphasia and exhibited word-retrieval difficulties. The clinical interview revealed that before retiring, this gentleman had worked in the men's clothing industry for many years. His face lit up whenever we brought up the topic of his work. The clinicians brought in pictures of shirts and ties, and asked him to identify and describe each item. They then went on to have the client coordinate various ensembles of these items, in pictures, and to discuss them. Given the opportunity to apply his area of expertise, the client developed his strength, enjoyed the activity, and his word-retrieval ability improved significantly.

Once we identify and understand an individual's strengths, we can strategize more effectively on how to address his weaknesses. Imagine that a child has difficulty understanding geometric concepts; however, the child is a strong artist. Instead of harping on his trouble with geometry, we might have the child draw a landscape scene. We may then ask him to divide the scene into geometric shapes and perpendicular lines. Finally, we might discuss the landscape using the target vocabulary.

Buckingham and Clifton (2001) pointed out that we grow the most and the fastest in our areas of strength and the least and slowest in our areas of weakness. That said, it is interesting that society encourages us to spend more time "fixing" what is deficient (Buckingham & Clifton, 2001). Further, if we ask someone to name his strengths, he may seem to be at a loss. On the other hand, if we ask the same individual to name his weaknesses, it becomes evident that he knows exactly what his weaknesses are (Ball, 2014; Buckingham & Clifton, 2001). When it comes to naming strengths, we must be aware of different cultural points of view. For example, a client of mine (BTA) hesitated to name her achievements because in her religious practice, talking about one's strengths was taboo and represented a lack of humility. Many of my (CSR) students and clients view discussing their own strengths as bragging.

Buckingham and Clifton (2001) highlighted their point about society's focus on weakness with the following example. They asked readers to imagine receiving their child's report card with the following grades:

- English: B
- Social Studies: B
- Art: A
- Science: B–
- Math: C

Which grade do you suppose gets the most attention? Probably, the C in math. According to Buckingham, most parents would focus on the weakest grade, even though more is accomplished by focusing on the strongest—the A in art. Math probably isn't this child's forte; however, art is his strong suit. Although math is a requirement and needs to be learned, the child could get support in math, and the school and parents could nurture his talent in art. One possible suggestion for building the child's confidence might be to ask each family member to write down a situation in which they observed the child display a unique strength. The family may then work together to create a "portrait" of the child that highlights his theme of inherent talents (Cameron, 2002).

When a child's grades do not meet the expectations of a parent, the teacher, or any other specialists working with the child (e.g., school speech-language pathologist, psychologist, guidance counselor) may call the speech-language pathologist. This becomes an opportunity for the clinician to work with the parent and child to recognize and develop strengths and to discuss the strategies needed to address his weaknesses. The following are several ways that a clinician may collaborate as part of a team to facilitate a child's poor or declining grades:

- Review the child's progress reports, report cards, and standardized test scores.
- Investigate the physical environment (seating, lighting, and noise).
- Discuss the course subject matter and whether the child understands the material.
- Ask the child how he would like to be helped.
- Look over the child's class notes.
- Help organize the child's backpack.
- Work out a daily schedule for studying that also allows time to pursue talents and interests (Box 7-2).

Box 7-2

A fifth grader who was having difficulty with academic demands was brought to my (BTA) office for an evaluation. During the clinical interview, I learned that this child loved to

(continued)

Box 7-2 (continued)

dance and that she attended ballet classes twice weekly. Her test results revealed below average performance in the areas of reading comprehension and word retrieval. After the evaluation, the mother explained that the father believed his daughter needed to stop her dance classes and to do her schoolwork independently. I explained that physical exercise can enhance a child's learning and attention. These improvements tend to raise the child's self-esteem (Ben-Shahar, 2010; Dawson & Guare, 2009). I further explained that it would be essential to provide her with language therapy. The parents decided to follow these recommendations, and as a result, their daughter continued with her dance classes and attended therapy sessions without resisting additional support. Over the course of the year her grades improved.

The father's solution to the situation in Box 7-2 was originally more punitive. He would have chosen to remove dance from his daughter's life because he thought it was time consuming and distracting. After realizing that this attitude would have brought his child into a downward cycle, the parents decided to incorporate what their daughter loved with her academic support system. By focusing on what a child can do well, she may become more competent, receptive, and willing to work on areas of weakness. As we will see later in this chapter, Fredrickson (2001) explained that an emotion such as joy can create an upward spiral of well-being, which generally helps a person reach her goal.

In positive psychology, *flow*, also known as *the zone,* is the state of mind a person experiences when performing an activity and is fully engaged, energized, focused, and at one with the activity. Some examples of flow would be an artist immersed in his painting, a ballerina involved in her dance, a runner experiencing a *runners high,* a speech-language pathologist involved in a counseling session, or a presenter or instructor delivering an engaging lecture (Csikszentmihalyi, 2008; Box 7-3).

Box 7-3

A 12-year-old boy was accompanied to my (CSR) office by his mother, who was concerned about her son's language and literacy difficulties. His mother entered the diagnostic room in a long coat, presented with a stooped posture, lowered head position, dark glasses, and a brimmed hat over her eyes. It appeared as though she was attempting to hide. During the interview, his mother persistently complained about her son's limitations. Her narrative consisted of describing her struggle over her son's failure to read books, his resistance to completing his homework, and his overall "laziness." I allowed the mother time to vent, to feel heard, and to feel validated (listening and empathy).

After a while, I requested her permission to ask a question. I asked her, "What do you see as your son's strengths, skills, or talents?" She answered immediately with a long list of attributes including the fact that he was kind, compassionate, and caring. The mother observed that he was the only one of her three children who ran out to carry in her packages or groceries. The mother went on to say that her son was a very loyal and devoted friend and that the other children loved him. In addition, he was an artist and a sculptor, who had recently won a prize for a piece of his artwork. I acknowledged how impressive

(continued)

Box 7-3 (CONTINUED)

her child was and how wonderfully in tune she was to his strengths and gifts. Now all she needed was the language to express this to her child.

All of a sudden, it appeared that a light bulb had turned on for this parent as she sat up taller, held her head higher, and maintained eye contact during this next interchange. She exclaimed, "Oh, I see…My relationship with my son has always been about telling him what he does wrong. I have never spoken to him about what he does well. You have changed my relationship with my son. From this day forward, our relationship will be different."

When I asked the mother the question about her son's strengths, my query came from a genuine curiosity rather than from a critical or judgmental place. The clinician's attitude, tone of voice, and sensitive choice of words impacts the way a client responds. The mother had all the wisdom and potential; she just needed a guide to bring these qualities out. Whether we agree with the parent or not, it is crucial we remember that empathy and listening must come first. We also need to trust that the parent is naturally creative, resourceful, and whole and has the ability to come to his own conclusions about his own life. By helping the parent access his own idea for a solution, the parent is more likely to own the idea and to follow through on these solutions.

Ask Yourself

As therapists, we are always trying to determine how to use a client's strength to address his weakness. Write three examples of weaknesses in your client and a way to address each by using the client's strengths.

Strengths and Feedback

Do you remember the last time someone paid you a compliment? Do you recall the last time you were criticized? Which stuck with you more? We tend to reject or invalidate positive feedback and dwell on negative feedback (Ben-Shahar, 2010). We call this the *Velcro and Teflon effect*—negative experiences and comments stick to us like Velcro, while the positive slides right off of us as if we were coated in Teflon. It is important to keep this concept in mind when offering feedback to our clients.

Barbara Fredrickson (2001) discovered that to thrive, individuals need a *3:1 ratio* of positive to negative experiences. Therefore, whenever we give negative feedback to a client, coworker, family member, or friend, we need to offer three positives to counter the one negative. Just as giving positive feedback is central to increasing the self-esteem of our clients, we need to change our negative self-talk to incorporate a 3:1 ratio within ourselves as well.

Although people need more positive than negative feedback, our clients come to us to improve their weaknesses. It is therefore important to offer our clients constructive support. The goal is to deliver these comments with sensitivity. When you give a client constructive feedback (the "1" in the 3:1 ratio), you build his trust. In time, he'll come to trust in your honesty and reliability. Bear in mind that the 3:1 ratio is an average and refers to a proportion, rather than to a fixed number.

Delivering Constructive Feedback

It has been our clinical experience that *constructive feedback* includes both the pros and cons of an individual's efforts. When providing constructive feedback, we suggest incorporating several important aspects and steps, including an introduction to the conversation, acknowledgment of the recipient, observations, suggestions for the future, and a take-away from the interaction. The following are some examples of constructive feedback adapted from Krenek (2012):

Step 1: State the Purpose of Your Feedback

Briefly explain the purpose for the conversation so that the receiver understands the agenda.

Instructor/Student: Let's go over your test results so that we can see where you had trouble and how you may improve.

Supervisor/Student: Let's talk today about providing client feedback.

Clinician/Parent: Let me tell you a little bit about what this session will look like.

Clinician/Client: Yesterday we worked on easy speech for words, and today we're going to work on easy speech for sentences.

Step 2: Acknowledge the Recipient

Acknowledgment is a powerful relationship builder.

Instructor/Student: I have found your contributions in class to be helpful to everyone.

Supervisor/Student: I like the way you reinforced Jimmy's production of "s" in a context other than the specific drill.

Clinician/Parent: I admire your courage and determination in the way you advocate for your child.

Clinician/Child: You really aced the way you made that "r" word. Let's see if we can get a few others.

Step 3: Observations

Observations refer to anything that the facilitator, student, parent, or client noticed or thought of in a clinical interaction. First, we recommend asking recipients what they noticed before telling them our observations. Notice the wording in the last two examples. This is called the *yes and tool.*

Instructor/Student: What can you tell me about Mary's strengths from her presentation?

Supervisor/Student: How did you feel when you were in that situation with the child?

Clinician/Parent: After observing your child's performance, what did you notice?…Yes, I agree with your observations and I also noticed…

Clinician/Client: After listening to the tape of your voice what are your thoughts about what you heard? Yes, I agree with you, and I also heard…

Step 4: Offer Specific Suggestions

Our suggestions ought to be helpful, practical, and include specific examples.

Instructor/Student: Before you are notified about the next exam, try working with a student who is strong in this topic, such as Mary or Bill.

Supervisor/Student: The next time you meet with this parent, try asking him about his son's strengths and interests.

Clinician/Parent: To help raise your daughter's self-esteem, try having each family member sit with her for 5 minutes a day and talk or engage in an activity.

Clinician/Client: The next time you are with a safe person, try talking to him about your speaking difficulties.

Step 5: Take-Away

At the conclusion of a class, clinical session, or counseling session with a parent and/or client, try asking the other individual a question such as, "What is one take-away you have from today's session?" An alternative way of asking this question is, "What did you learn from today's session?" (Krenek, 2012).

Constructive Feedback for Children

Children receive daily feedback from their parents and teachers. The feedback may be in the form of general and/or exaggerated praise for their achievements and/or talents. It may be verbal or written such as on an exam or report card. The feedback may be delivered in the form of general criticism for less-than-perfect grades or expressions of disappointment. This combination of commentary and/or grades may be confusing to the child, who always expects success as well, as compared to the child who generally achieves low grades. A child who receives high grades may feel like a failure when he is unsuccessful, and the child who generally receives lower grades may become resigned to failure. This type of commentary perpetuates a faltering self-esteem and weakened self-confidence (Dweck, 2006).

Dweck (2006) recommended focusing on the child's learning *process* and the *effort* the child makes. It is essential to recognize the child's process and effort and provide the child with the tools needed to achieve his goals. For example, a child may inform a parent about a good grade he received on an exam. To focus on the process and effort the child made, the parent may then ask about the amount of time he studied, how he analyzed the material, how he prepared for the test, and how he feels about his achievement. On the other hand, for the child who comes home disappointed in his grade, we need to be mindful about judging and making negative comments. We must lean into the child's strengths and into what the child may do to better succeed. An effective question might be, "What do you think you need to get to the next step?" It is important to note the effort by saying something like, "I know you tried very hard." In this way, parents, teachers, clinical supervisors, clinicians, and administrators may instill a love of learning, increase resilience, and serve as role models of this love, passion, enthusiasm, and excitement for their clients and students (Box 7-4).

Box 7-4

Recently, a 6-year-old boy with a repaired cleft lip and palate entered the therapy room excited about how he had been doing as a member of the chess club at his school. I (BTA) listened carefully and then asked him how he had been managing to do everything from chess to soccer and still complete his speech work. He described his learning and practice. I commented that his efforts were admirable. He asked what the meaning of effort was and accepted my explanation. As he tackled the next group of words during our session, he stopped and asked, "Is this effort?" This child engaged in the process of discussion related to his effort and goals. He now keeps a little note in his homework book that says, "Effort and patience lead to success."

Ask Yourself

1. Where in your clinical work or teaching might you have overlooked the 3:1 ratio?

2. Write about a situation where you could use the 3:1 ratio with a client.

3. Describe a situation in which you were disappointed with the feedback you received. Write which of the five steps of constructive feedback were included and which were omitted.

4. Describe a situation in which your feedback may have focused on the result rather than on the process and the effort. What could you have said alternatively?

LABELING DIMINISHES STRENGTH

Despite the proven importance of assuming a strengths perspective, as speech-language pathologists trained in the medical model, we tend to group our clients under generic labels, and most likely, we do the same to ourselves. How often have you heard someone say, "I am definitely ADHD (attention-deficit/hyperactivity disorder)," or "I am certain that I have an auditory processing disorder." That kind of self-deprecation assumes a deficits perspective, strips our clients of individuality, and turns the speaker into the problem he has named. For example, if one who stutters becomes "the stutterer," the human being is lost to a label (Davis, 2004). To that end, in a recent excerpt on the *Today* show, a mother spoke about her daughter's blindness as follows: "She is not blindness; she is our beautiful little girl who happens to be blind." Similarly, in our profession we choose not to identify a child by a label, such as "autistic," "cognitively challenged," "deaf," "stutterer," etc. We would rather say a "child who has autism," "a person who stutters," or one who has a hearing loss.

The Social Model of Disabilities

When we emphasize a deficit, it affects not only how we view our clients, but how we interact with them as well; it generates a self-fulfilling prophecy or self-limiting belief, which reveals how labels disable. The social model of disability maintains that society, not the person with a disability, is the disabled party. This model emphasizes the importance of altering society's perspective rather than striving to "fix" the client (Michigan Disabilities Rights Coalition Social Model of Disabilities, n.d.). Kathie Snow eloquently summarizes this perspective in the following:

> Nothing short of a paradigm shift in how we think about disability is necessary for change to occur. Disability, like ethnicity, religion, age, gender, and other characteristics, is a natural part of life. Some people are born with disabilities and some acquire them later in life. (And if we live long enough, many of us will acquire a disability through an accident, illness, or the aging process.)

> A disability label is not the defining characteristic of a person, any more than one's age, religion, ethnicity, or gender is the defining characteristic. We must never use a disability label to measure a person's value or predict a person's potential, and we must recognize that the presence of a disability is not an inherent barrier to a person's success.

> We do not need to change people with disabilities! We need to change ourselves, and how we think about disability. When we think differently, we'll talk differently. When we think and talk differently, we'll act differently. When we act differently, we'll be creating change in ourselves, and our communities. In the process, the lives of people with disabilities will be changed, as well.

> Reprinted with permission from Snow, K. (2007). Counseling in communication disorders: A wellness perspective. San Diego, CA: Plural Publishing Inc.

Solution-Focused Brief Therapy

We'd to like to introduce a counseling model that incorporates all of the tools, skills, and attitudes that we have discussed thus far. This approach to counseling is strengths-based and referred to as *SFBT, brief therapy*, or *solution-focused therapy*. These terms are used interchangeably. SFBT has been empirically proven in the literature to be effective in a wide variety of helping professions and to be a short-term form of treatment. As you continue to read, you will learn that this approach provides excellent tools for the speech-language pathologist and audiologist to supplement their clinical interactions with clients and families (Ouelette, 2004).

The SFBT model allows the client to co-create with the clinician and a vision for the future. This approach also helps to facilitate finding new ways to manage difficulties. SFBT increases client and family confidence and empowers them to be agents of change (Ouellette, 2004). The model provides hope and confidence that clinicians, clients, and families have the tools to handle crises. Using a coaching approach, with an emphasis on deep empathic listening and specific language, the SFBT clinician prioritizes linking the present with the future, which helps the client move forward (Burns, 2006).

The medical model of telling and advising is problem and clinician focused, delivers content, advises, labels, and does not focus on feelings. On the other hand, SFBT emphasizes the emotional component of the challenge, trusts in the client and family's resource-fulness, creativity, and in the ability for the client and clinician to establish a co-creative relationship (partnership).

At the onset of a diagnostic session, the opening questions, according to the medical model might be, "When did the problem first begin?" "What are the symptoms?" and so on. The SFBT approach focuses on what's working and/or what the client has done well. Based on the medical model, the clinician might ask the question, "What brought you here today?" where the focus is on the problem and requires a lengthy description of the negative. An SFBT opening question would sound more like, "How can I be useful to you today?" which focuses more on the construction of solutions (Ouellette, 2004). According to Burns (2006), "The shift toward constructing solutions to problems, rather than deconstructing the problem, is the fundamental difference between SFBT and a problem-solving approach."

Speech-language pathologists have recently begun to incorporate the SFBT approach for their clients with a range of speech, language, and communication difficulties (Burns, 2006; Cook & Botterill, 2009; Ouellette, 2004). This technique is used extensively at the Michael Palin Centre for Stammering in England. Clinicians may use this approach with young children as long as the children are mature enough to understand the questions. In addition, SFBT intervention has been shown to have therapeutic effects to enhance the self-esteem of students (Taathadi, 2014).

We as speech-language pathologists and audiologists, who tend to limit ourselves to a problem-solving approach to fix what is broken, may better serve our clients by expanding our approach to include a client- and family-centered model (Geller & Foley, 2009) such as SFBT. The following will clarify how to conduct an SFBT session.

Solution-Focused Brief Therapy: Sequence of an Initial Session

An SFBT session may include the following components: adversity, best hopes (goal), exceptions to the rule, exception that proves the rule, miracle question, scaling, and ending the session. It is important to note that the clinician need not apply all of the parts described in this sequence. It is up to the clinician to select the appropriate segment(s) according to the client's needs, the nature of the problem, timing (where you are in a conversation), and time constraints.

Adversity

The clinician establishes the issue, or the reason the client has come to the session. The first question might be, "How can I be useful to you today?" or "How will you know this session has been useful to you?" or "What will it take for you to say that this meeting has been worthwhile?" (Burns, 2006). These first questions lead us to the next segment.

Best Hopes (Goal)

Best hopes refers to a short- or long-term goal. For example, the client's best hopes may be that he wants more confidence, to improve communication in social situations, or to have a more pleasant sounding voice. In SFBT, the clinician guides the client to decide what he wants to take away from the evaluation or therapy, thereby shifting the responsibility to the client to make his own decisions and to find his own solutions. Once the client articulates the goal, the facilitator asks additional strength-based questions. For example, if a client says he would like to feel "more confident interacting with others," the clinician might ask, "How will you know when you are more confident?" The client would then explain what he does differently when he is "more confident." For example, the client might say, "When I'm confident, I speak up more in front of a group."

Next, the clinician summarizes in writing what the client has said and then asks, "Who else will notice that you are more confident?" and "What difference will that make to those people?" The client may respond, "My colleagues will notice that I'm more participatory in group discussions."

One powerful question that helps the client add to his list of stated goals is, "What else?" We use the phrase, "What else?" rather than, "Anything else?" because the former phrase is open-ended and assumes that the client has more information. The latter phrase is a closed-ended "yes–no" question, which is limiting.

Exceptions to the Rule

It is the job of the instructor or clinician to point out exceptions to the rule, or the times the client does better, for example, when he shows increased confidence or reduced stuttering, which is a sign of progress. The key is to highlight for him that an exception need not be an isolated occurrence; if it happened once, it can happen again. Scientists have demonstrated that past behavior predicts future performance (Ouellette & Wood, 1998). By encouraging the client to glimpse his preferred future, we show him it is possible to achieve and succeed in similar ways in the present and future.

As speech-language pathologists who work with children with specific oral motor and articulation difficulties, we know that therapy can become frustrating for the client as well as the clinician. Yet when the client unexpectedly produces the targeted change (e.g., the correct phoneme), we get a peek into what is possible; we see the pathway to future progress. We may say to the client, "Once is just the beginning."

The Exception Proves the Rule

In the 1950s, when Roger Bannister, a competitive runner, broke the 4-minute mile barrier by running a 3.9-minute mile, he taught us that the exception proves the rule. As a result, Bannister created a self-fulfilling prophecy. Other elite runners saw that there was no longer a boundary; they too could do what Bannister had done. Soon runners all over the world were matching Bannister's time and then beating it. By finding the exception to the rule of our problems and crises, we develop confidence that we are already *there*, that we have touched success and glimpsed the miracle (Ben-Shahar, 2010; Box 7-5).

Box 7-5

A client came to my (CSR) office struggling with shyness and social anxiety. The following excerpt is the SFBT conversation that we had.

- **Question:** What would you like to focus on this session?
  - **Response:** I have been really shy my whole life. Lately, I feel like it gets in the way of my functioning.
- **Question:** Are there any times when you feel less shy or more outgoing?
  - **Response:** Yes.
- **Question:** What are you doing when you feel less shy or more outgoing? Can you think of examples from the recent past?
  - **Response:** Well, this week at a wedding, I bumped into some old friends from high school. It was very exciting to see them again.
- **Question:** Tell me more about that.
  - **Response:** We reminisced about the old days, recalled some inside jokes, and laughed a lot.
- **Question:** So you enjoyed being with people who knew you well. You felt comfortable, had some good laughs, and rekindled old relationships. What was that like for you? What did you do to behave in an outgoing way? What did that look like?
  - **Response:** I felt free and able to be myself. I did not worry about sounding dumb or uninteresting. Everyone responded to what I had to say. I felt alive. I guess I smiled and laughed a lot, I asked them a lot of questions, just let myself go!

Ask Yourself

These questions may give you greater access to your goal.

- When do you feel most confident?

- Where do you feel most confident?

- Who is around you when you are feeling most confident?

- What do you notice about yourself when you are confident?

- What else do you notice? (Adapted from Burns, 2006)

- Give examples of an SFBT interaction involving a client's story. How would this apply to someone in your case load?

The Miracle Question

To obtain more information about the client's preferred future and what is important to him, we present what Greenberger and Padesky (1995) call the *miracle question*. The miracle question requires that the client visualizes his preferred future. We ask the client to picture that his difficulty has been completely resolved. We might phrase it like this: "Imagine that someone waved a magic wand while you were asleep, and when you woke up, your problem was gone." We ask the client to imagine he no longer stutters or no longer suffers the effects of his stroke—that his speech is clear and articulate. "What difference would that make in your life?" we ask. After some thought, the client usually responds with a clear and detailed picture of his preferred future.

Scaling Questions

Scaling questions help us apply a numerical representation to strengths. Once we assign a number (0 to 10 or some variation), we have chosen a goal to strive for. Scaling questions help us to stop thinking of ourselves in absolutes, perfect or failing, and instead help us see ourselves on a continuum. Furthermore, the scales are used to gain an understanding of the family's perspective, motivate and encourage clients, uncover exceptions to obstacles, visually note progress, and develop goals (Berg & de Shazer, 1993; Cade & O'Hanlon, 1993; Franklin, Corcoran, Nowicki, & Streeter, 1997; Selekman, 1997). The specific numbers are not that relevant, so whatever the individual puts down on the scale is accepted at face value. The most important part of scaling comes in the questions that follow. Scaling questions, such as, "On a scale from 0 to 10, where 0 is worst and 10 is best, how will you know when you are at a 9?" or "What difference will that make?" are useful for everything from sparking motivation, to building confidence, to self-assessing a skill.

Now turn your attention to a sample scaling dialogue between clinician and client (Boxes 7-6 and 7-7).

Box 7-6

SAMPLE SCALING QUESTIONS

- How have you managed to get to a 5?
- How will you know when you are at an 8?
- What are you doing differently when you are at an 8?
- How will you know things are going well?
- What difference will that make to you?
- Who else will notice?
- What difference will that make to them?
- What else?

Once again, write down the client's information so that he may review this with the clinician.

Box 7-7

SCALING SAMPLE

- **Clinician:** On a scale from 0 to 10, where 0 is worst and 10 is the best, what number is your confidence right now?
  - **Client:** I would say about a 3.
- **Clinician:** So, in terms of how outgoing you are, your number is 3. How did you manage to get to a 3?
  - **Client:** I guess there are times when I feel more confident talking, like when I'm speaking to family members or close friends.
- **Clinician:** And on a scale from 0 to 10, where 0 is worst and 10 is best, what number would be good enough for you as your ultimate goal?
  - **Client:** I think that if I could bring my confidence up to an 8, that would be good enough.
- **Clinician:** An 8. Wonderful! Let's mark that on the scale. What would you be doing differently at an 8 than you're doing at a 3?
  - **Client:** At an 8, I would be smiling and laughing a lot more and looking straight at people, rather than looking down. People tell me I look down a lot.
- **Clinician:** So at an 8, you would be making more eye contact and acting happier. (Clinician writes this down on the pad.)
- **Clinician:** And if you were making eye contact, smiling, and laughing more, what difference would that make to you?

(continued)

Box 7-7 (CONTINUED)

- ○ **Client:** I would feel free, like a weight had been lifted from me. I would not worry about what I was saying or how I was saying it. I would just be in the moment with people; I'd be engaged, interested, and happy to feel connected.

- **Clinician:** Excellent. Let's write down those feelings you just described. (The clinician writes the summary in his client's words on a pad.)

- **Clinician:** And who else would notice?

- ○ **Client:** Well, my friends; all the people I am with would notice. Even people in the room who are not speaking directly to me would notice my confidence level.

- **Clinician:** What would they notice about you?

- ○ **Client:** They would notice how confident I look, how comfortable I am in my own skin, and that I hold myself and move in a carefree manner. (Clinician writes all these points down and reviews them with his client.)

- **Clinician:** And what difference would that make to them?

- ○ **Client:** My friends and acquaintances would find it easier to talk to me. I would be a person they'd seek out because they'd see how free and relaxed I am. They would want to be around me because our time together would be fun and full of laughter.

- **Clinician:** And what else?

- ○ **Client:** My phone would ring with invitations. People would want to get together with me for dinner, drinks, and movies. They would invite me to their parties and gatherings. I would have an active social life. (The clinician writes all these observations down on the shared pad so that his client could see his preferred future.)

- **Clinician:** So, over the course of the week, at one major event, you were feeling pretty outgoing and friendly and weren't second-guessing yourself. You were being you! That's fabulous!

Ending the Session

As critical as it is to set the tone at the beginning of the session, it's equally important to end the session on a hopeful note and with a feeling of accomplishment. We want the client to leave with a concrete goal (Box 7-8).

Box 7-8

SAMPLE FEEDBACK TO END THE SESSION

Clinician: I'm really impressed with how you broke out of your shell at the party. Parties can be intimidating. The fact that you let yourself go and enjoyed the moment speaks to your potential to be more confident; you're already doing it! Since you brought up this party today, what might be a good follow-up goal for next week?

(continued)

Box 7-8 (CONTINUED)

Client: Hmmm, I'm not sure…

Clinician: May I offer a suggestion?

Client: Of course!

Clinician: How about over the course of the week, you jot down at least one situation in which you noticed yourself breaking the status quo by being more outgoing and less self-conscious. Will you let me know about that next week?

Client: Sure!

Clinician: How will you let me know (phone, text, email, or in person)?

Ask Yourself

Engage in a discussion with a friend.

1. Take turns telling each other all of the evidence you've noticed since you woke up this morning that it's good to be alive. Then, together, review the effects of doing this exercise (Cook & Botterill, 2009).

2. Choose what you consider to be the strength that is most *you*. Try to apply this strength in a situation to which you've never applied it before. Record the results (Seligman, 2002).

3. Find at least one classmate who shares your signature strength. Discuss how you each use and manifest it in your everyday lives. Compare and brainstorm new ways to apply your strength (Seligman, 2002).

4. Engage in an SFBT session with your buddy. Take turns being the client and clinician. Choose a challenging situation, past or future. Remember the sequence of the program as follows:

   a. Adversity: clarify the reason the client came to you

   b. Best hopes: clarify the goal

   c. Exceptions to the rule

   d. Miracle question

   e. Scale the goal

   f. Review the scale on a shared sheet of paper, recording the client's observations and comments.

   g. Provide feedback and be sure to acknowledge your client for their effort.

KEY CONCEPTS

- Positive psychologists emphasize the importance of focusing on strengths, rather than weaknesses.
- Society emphasizes weakness.
- Use weaknesses to address strengths.
- Fredrickson's (2001) 3:1 ratio means three positive comments to counteract one negative.

- Steps for delivering constructive feedback include: purpose, acknowledgment, observation, suggestions, and take-away.

- Social model of disabilities emphasizes that society's perspective and behavior toward individuals with disabilities must be altered.

- Labeling is disabling.

- Positive psychologists assembled a manual of 24 strengths that are ubiquitous among human beings.

- Although we are not psychologists, we must be equipped to address normal human struggle such as a communication disorder.

- SFBT is solution focused.

- SFBT integrates listening and language and links the present to the possible future.

- A comparison between a client and family centered approach (e.g., SFBT) and a clinician-focused approach, such as the medical model is discussed.

- An SFBT session may include any one or a combination of the following segments: adversity, best hopes, exceptions to the rule, exception that proves the rule, miracle question, and scaling.

REFERENCES

Ball, R. (2014) *Being with*. Bloomington, IN: Author House.

Ben-Shahar, T. (2010). *Foundations of positive psychology* [PowerPoint slides]. Retrieved from www.slideshare.net/dadalaolang/1504-01intro?ref=http://positivepsychologyprogram.com/harvard-positive-psychology-course

Berg, I. K., & de Shazer, S. (1993). *Making numbers talk: Language in therapy*. In S. Freidman (Ed.), *The new language of change*. New York, NY: Guilford Press.

Buckingham, M., & Clifton, D. O. (2001). *Now, discover your strengths*. New York, NY: Simon & Schuster.

Burns, K. (2006). *Focus on solutions: A health professional's guide*. Hoboken, NJ: John Wiley & Sons.

Cade, B., & O'Hanlon, W. H. (1993). *A brief guide to brief therapy*. New York, NY: W.W. Norton.

Cameron, J. (2002). *The artist's way*. Westminster, United Kingdom: Penguin Books.

Cook, F., & Botterill, W. (2009). *Tools for success: A cognitive behavioral therapy taster* [DVD]. Boston, MA: Stuttering Foundation of America.

Csikszentmihalyi, M. (2008). *Flow: The psychology of optimal experience*. New York, NY: Harper Perennial.

Davis, K. (2004). What's in a name: Our only label should be our name: Avoiding the stereotypes. *The Reporter, 9*(2), 10-12, 24.

Dawson, P., & Guare, R. (2009). *Smart but scattered: The revolutionary "executive skills" approach to helping kids reach their potential*. New York, NY: Guilford Press.

de Shazer, S. (1988). *Clues: Investigating solutions in brief therapy*. New York, NY: W.W. Norton.

Dweck, C. (2006). *Mindset*. New York: Random House.

Franklin, C., Corcoran, J., Nowicki, J., & Streeter, C. (1997). Using client self-anchored scales to measure outcomes in solution-focused therapy. *Journal of Systemic Therapies, 16*, 246–265.

Fredrickson, B. L. (2001). The role of positive emotions in positive psychology: The broaden-and-build theory of positive emotions. *American Psychologist, 56*(3), 218–226.

Geller, E., & Foley, G. M. (2009). Broadening the "ports of entry" for speech-language pathologists: A relational and reflective model for clinical supervision. *American Journal of Speech-Language Pathology, 18*(1), 22–41.

Greenberger, D., & Padesky, C. A. (1995). *Mind over mood: Change how you feel by changing the way you think*. New York, NY: Guilford Press.

Holland, A. L. (2007). *Counseling in communication disorders: A wellness perspective*. San Diego, CA: Plural.

Krenek, C. (2012). How to give constructive feedback in 6 easy steps [Web log post]. Retrieved from http://info.profilesinternational.com/profiles-employee-assessment-blog/bid/102602/How-To-Give-Constructive-Feedback-in-6-Easy-Steps

Michigan Disability Rights Coalition. (n.d.). Definition 2. *Models of Disability*. Retrieved from www.copower.org/leadership/models-of-disability

Ouellette, S. E. (2004). Clinical issues: Applications of solution-focused concepts to the practice of speech-language pathology. *SIG 1 Perspectives on Language Learning and Education, 11*(1), 8–14.

Ouellette, J. A., & Wood, W. (1998). Habit and intention in everyday life: The multiple processes by which past behavior predicts future behavior. *Psychological Bulletin, 124*(1), 54.

Peterson, C., & Seligman, M. E. (2004). *Character strengths and virtues: A handbook and classification.* New York, NY: Oxford University Press.

Selekman, M. D. (1997). *Solution-focused therapy with children: Harnessing family strengths for systemic change.* New York, NY: Guilford Press.

Seligman, M. E., & Peterson, C. (2002). *Authentic happiness: Using the new positive psychology to realize your potential for lasting fulfillment.* New York, NY: Free Press.

Snow, K. (2007). *Counseling in communication disorders: A wellness perspective.* San Diego, CA: Plural Publishing Inc

Taathadi, M. S. (2014). Application of solution-focused brief therapy (SFBT) to enhance high school students self-esteem: An embedded experimental design. *International Journal of Psychological Studies, 6*(3), 96–105.

RECOMMENDED WEBSITES

Keirsey: http://keirsey.com
Clifton StrengthsFinder: www.strengthsfinder.com
University of Pennsylvania, Authentic Happiness: www.authentichappiness.org
StandOut: www.marcusbuckingham.com

8

Raising Resilience

In the depth of winter, I finally learned that within me there lay an invincible summer.

—Albert Camus, 1970

LEARNER OUTCOMES

After reading this chapter, the reader will be able to:

1. Identify and describe the components of resilience according to Reivich and Shatté.

2. Cite five strategies, according to the Intentional Resilience Center, to develop resilience.

3. Distinguish among adversities, thoughts, and emotions.

4. Describe the realistic optimism–pessimism continuum, including negative thinking styles.

5. Describe how narrative therapy builds resilience.

6. Complete a resilience grid (ABCD) according to the cognitive model on *self* and *other*.

Victor Frankl, an early positive psychologist who survived the Holocaust, was the first to examine resilience in the face of adversity. In his book, *Man's Search for Meaning* (1985), Frankl highlights one of the most powerful examples of resilience—the ability of some of the prisoners to remain strong in the face of unbearable circumstances. Through his observations, Frankl came to the conclusion that the survivors' ability to alter their perspective about their horrific experiences and their capacity to derive meaning from them were foundational to their resilience and survival. Frankl made meaning out of his catastrophic circumstances by visualizing, in great detail, how he would lecture his students about what he had endured and survived (Nourse, 2015).

Stein-Rubin, C., & Adler, B. T. *Counseling in Communication Disorders: Facilitating the Therapeutic Rehabilitation* (pp 125-140).

People handle adversity in a variety of ways. For some, life is a war, and every day is a battle—they *catastrophize* (Burns, 1999), or magnify, their everyday obstacles. On the other end of the spectrum, some people, in the face of difficult life circumstances, bounce back better and stronger than before. This powerful quality is called *resilience*, which is the ability to overcome major obstacles, steer through the trials and tribulations of everyday life, bounce back from adversity, and reach out of one's comfort zone (Reivich & Shatté, 2002). Resilience increases happiness, well-being, and self-esteem and is an essential ingredient in dealing with our fast-paced, overwhelming, and highly stressful world. Resilience can help us in all facets of life, including our education, careers, work–life balance, and relationships.

Why do some individuals succeed regardless of dire circumstances? In a study of Vietnam War prisoners who did not suffer from post-traumatic stress disorder, researchers investigated the qualities that helped these heroes survive despite unbearable circumstances. Resilience was a key factor (Reivich & Shatté, 2002).

Many people think of resilience as the ability to recover from difficult life circumstances, or the ability to manage the vicissitudes of everyday living; however, Reivich and Shatté's definition encompasses the four following factors:

1. Overcoming

2. Steering through

3. Bouncing back

4. Reaching out

The fourth component means that resilient individuals take risks despite their challenges, reach out of their comfort zones, and live out their potential. These individuals are not just living life and successfully overcoming adversity, they are flourishing.

Although much of a person's resilience is inborn, psychologists have proven that resilience can be taught (Burns, 1999; Greenberger & Padesky, 1995; Nourse, 2015; Reivich & Shatté, 2002). These experts have introduced and demonstrated how to apply the principles of resilience and flexible thinking to everyone. The good news is that if you are already resilient, you have the potential to become more resilient. If you aren't naturally resilient, you can develop this powerful quality. Most of us fall along a resilience continuum, rather than into an all or nothing category.

At the Penn State Resilience Programs, developed by Reivich and Shatté (2002), which works with both United States Army soldiers and late elementary and middle school students, they successfully teach core optimism and resilience skills. They prove that we can train individuals to be more resilient; it's all about modifying the way they think about adversity. As Aaron Beck, the father of cognitive behavioral therapy, said, "Men are disturbed not by things but by the view which they take of them" (Reivich & Shatté, 2002). In other words, it is not the problem, but the reaction to the problem, that is the enemy. We may not have choice about an existing adversity; however, we have choice about how we think about it, view it, and react to it; this requires flexible thinking.

According to the Intentional Resiliency Framework (Nourse, 2015), the six following strategies were found to build resilience:

1. *Develop support networks:* It is important to reach out to fellow professionals and individuals both inside and outside of your work environment.

2. *Clarify purpose:* It is important to visualize what may be accomplished once one has adapted to their adversity. Recall Chapter 7 on the importance of visualization in solution-focused brief therapy (SFBT).

3. *Build self-awareness:* Engage in mindfulness work and meditation, enroll in a self-awareness class, work with a life coach or therapist, register for a graduate-level counseling course, and read books on the topic (see suggested readings in the Appendix).

4. *Enhance self-care:* Our resiliency as clinicians and leaders depends on our physical and emotional well-being. For us to maintain our balance, remain centered, and maintain our resiliency, it is essential that we eat healthy, get enough sleep, exercise, and engage in some form of relaxation.

5. *Actualize strengths:* Resilient people are aware of what they excel in and know how to lean into those strengths (see Chapter 7). That is why these individuals tend to speak out more at meetings and have more self-confidence in presentations.

6. *Broaden coping strategies:* Rather than become stuck on the problem, resilient people reach out to others, develop a plan, create a vision, and find ways to modify negative perspectives.

As speech-language pathologists and audiologists, we interact daily with normal human beings going through the "full catastrophe" (Kingsley, 1987) of what it means to be human. Our clients and their families are handling the trials and tribulations of communication disorders. As helping professionals, we support the people we work with to gain access to greater hope and optimism—and consequently, to thrive and live fulfilling lives despite the obstacles. In this chapter, we provide counseling models, reflective work, and examples on how to develop our own resilience as clinicians and how to be role models for our clients and their families.

Ask Yourself

1. How have you chosen to move forward in a situation, despite your fear?

2. What did it take for you to take this step, and what was the outcome?

RESILIENCE IN PEOPLE WHO STUTTER

To illustrate all parts of Reivich and Shatté's (2002) definition (overcoming, bouncing back, steering through, and reaching out), we turn to persons who stutter (PWS). These individuals must overcome a life-altering obstacle; they often suffer consequences far broader than the observable disfluencies in their speech. Although research and treatment emphasize the behavioral features of stuttering, the psychological ramifications of this disorder (illustrated in Sheehan's [1970] iceberg metaphor; see Chapter 3) may be even more damaging. Stuttering can interfere with relationships, education, employment, personal expression, and self-esteem (Yaruss, 2010).

It has been found that resilient individuals have more methods of coping and putting themselves on the line than their less resilient peers. As shown by Sheehan's iceberg metaphor, some people who exhibit mild stuttering characteristics may have a significant emotional component as well. On the other hand, PWS who have significant stuttering characteristics may have mild emotional ramifications. As we have observed, the severity of the stuttering characteristics is not necessarily correlated to the extent of the emotional aspect of the disorder (Boxes 8-1 and 8-2).

Box 8-1

In 2011, I (CSR) conducted a workshop presentation at the Canadian Stuttering Association that focused on how resilience affects the educational and career choices of PWS. I was interested in the fact that the severity of external stuttering characteristics did not seem to predict situations, or even careers, PWS would choose. In fact, a PWS with severe stuttering characteristics chaired the event and introduced me to the audience. Often, PWS have remarkable courage; at the workshop, many reached out of their comfort zones and delivered speeches.

Box 8-2

Lazaro Arbos, a PWS who auditioned for *American Idol*, may have felt extreme pressure during his audition. Arbos struggled and used his hands to gesture in an attempt to get his words out. He had a tough time even saying his own name; nevertheless, he persevered, introduced himself and his song, and answered the judges' questions. When Lazaro sang, his performance was transformative—he had the voice of an angel. Arbos's stunning vocal rendition was not the only compelling element of his debut. PWS tend not to stutter when they sing, so when it came time for Arbos to sing, his chances of impressing the judges were about the same as anyone's. To us, the most inspiring part of the audition was that this young man, who stuttered so severely, had the courage to speak, and therefore to stutter, in front of millions of people. His story is the personification of resilience.

It has been our clinical experience that no correlation exists between the severity of someone's stutter and the degree to which she avoids speaking. Why is that? What makes one person push through a distracting speech pattern to pursue his dream, while another person with less overt challenges withdraws? This question provides further support for the ways resilience influences optimal support.

Ask Yourself

Think of an example of a person you know who suffers from a disability and reaches out of her comfort zone regardless of her special needs. Explain how your example fits Reivich and Shatté's definition of resilience.

As you progress through this chapter you will notice that two important aspects of resilience are realistic optimism and pessimism (Seligman, 2002) and flexible thinking styles (Reivich & Shatté, 2002).

REALISTIC OPTIMISM AND PESSIMISM

Seligman's (2002) definition of optimism does not suggest that we adopt a Pollyanna-type approach to life. He calls this *unrealistic optimism* and says it is as dangerous as pessimism. In other words, people who are unrealistically optimistic, who claim that everyone and everything is wonderful, may underestimate certain risks to their own health and safety. Seligman prefers *realistic optimism*. This is the ability to look honestly at what is, as well as what is possible, and to choose a perspective that enhances reality.

Negative Thinking Styles

Seligman (2002) teaches that we improve our resilience by becoming aware of our *thinking and interpretation styles* (the way we interpret events in our lives). We also improve our resilience by avoiding *default reactions* (we must be proactive rather than reactive) and *core beliefs* (learning our habitual ways of looking at the world) and challenging our *limiting beliefs* (negative thought patterns). He emphasizes the need to understand one's interpretation of what happens in life as part of a continuum. This continuum includes three components: *me vs not me* (accepting blame or placing it elsewhere), *something vs everything* ("I have a problem" vs "I have a terrible life"), or *sometimes vs always* (believing that life has ups and downs vs believing that the negatives are ever-present). These negative thinking styles may prevent flexible thinking, realistic optimism, and then may severely diminish one's resilience (Reivich & Shatté, 2002).

Psychologists such as Ben-Shahar (2010) teach us that our habitual optimistic vs pessimistic thought patterns actually change the form of our brains (transformation). We physically create our own positive and negative neural pathways by repeatedly engaging in the same types of thoughts. For example, if we have a pessimistic thinking style, we carve negative thinking pathways in our brains, which become deeper and neurologically light up more. These more established pathways are the places where our mind gravitates, becomes our default neurological reaction, and determines how we then create our reality.

Ask Yourself

Take a moment to think about where you are on the optimism–pessimism continuum. Mark an X on the line below where 0 represents the most pessimistic and 10 represents the most optimistic:

0_____10

(Adapted from Seligman, 2002.)

Learned Helplessness

Seligman's (2002) book *Authentic Happiness* teaches us that individuals who have had repeated exposure to frustrating and painful events as a result of a traumatic life circumstance may give up and retreat from persisting. He called this behavior *learned helplessness*. Learned helplessness may be applied to the clients we see in our caseload, such as with the PWS who has been bullied and withdraws from speaking; the individual with learning disabilities who, due to repeated failed attempts, no longer attempts to read; and the client with aphasia who has experienced repeated failure and humiliation when attempting to engage in conversation, and gives up as a result.

Narrative Therapy and Resilience

DiLollo, Manning, and Neimeyer (2003, 2005) have done important work regarding *narrative therapy*. The narrative model teaches us that people are *storytellers* and that their personal stories, or beliefs about themselves, determine the view they take of themselves in the context of their lives (Madigan & Goldner, 1998; Neimeyer, 1995; Winslade & Monk, 1999). This model corresponds to what we have just learned in Seligman's discussion of negative thinking styles and learned helplessness. Listening to clients' narratives is important in helping us clarify the events in the story and their sequence. Furthermore, as we listen to our clients' stories, we gain access to their self-concepts. The story a client tells about herself may become a self-fulfilling prophecy and consequently a recurring theme throughout her life. For example, the client who fears public speaking may build on those fears with each negative public speaking event, confirming her belief that she can't speak in front of groups.

When individuals tell their own stories they tend to describe themselves negatively, put themselves down, and then go on to develop a defeatist attitude (Stacey, 1997). It is part and parcel of our role to help direct our clients' stories in a more positive and truthful direction. As clinicians, we help to co-create clients' stories so that they are more helpful to the client (DiLollo & Neimeyer, 2014; Frid, Oehlen, & Bergbom, 2003). By empathizing, listening critically, and responding actively (reflecting, paraphrasing, clarifying, asking open-ended questions, and using clinical intuition), the clinician may help the client shift perspectives to a more realistic and adaptive one.

As speech-language pathologists and audiologists, we must also note that there will be times when we will notice that the client is invested in her narrative, and regardless of our efforts to co-construct, the client's resistance may be stronger. This situation may occur during the diagnostic evaluation or therapy. To maintain our ethical responsibility, and to prioritize the client's needs, it is essential for us to acknowledge that the problem may be more deeply rooted than it first appeared to be and may be outside of our scope of practice. If this is the case, we discuss the situation with the client, and then make the recommendation for additional support with a professional who may have greater expertise in this area (Box 8-3).

Box 8-3

A 3-year-old child who presented with severely delayed speech and language was seen at my (CSR) office. During the evaluation, it quickly became apparent that he exhibited behavioral and emotional issues. At one point, the sky darkened, and it began to rain lightly. Terrified, the child began to cry and scream; it was difficult to calm him down. During the post-evaluation conference, I asked his mother what she noticed about her child's behavior. She noted that he was difficult to control, anxious, fearful, a bully at home and in class, and that today's behavior was typical.

The parent also observed that some of the techniques used during the session, such as turning tasks into games, using positive reinforcement, and providing choices for activities, were helpful in eliciting more positive responses. I acknowledged her observations and asked her permission to make a suggestion to which she responded positively. We discussed a treatment plan that would also include the additional support of a behavioral counselor to address her concerns about her child's behavior. She was assured that the speech-language pathologist would work closely with her and the behavioral counselor to facilitate her child's progress.

In the case of therapeutic intervention, one may encounter a client who has struggled with the same limiting beliefs for an extended period of time (Box 8-4).

Box 8-4

A teenager who stutters was seen at my (BTA) office over a period of several months. She maintained a pessimistic thinking style and believed that, despite her significant progress in school, at home, and socially, she was dysfluent all the time. One day when the client appeared to be sad and frustrated about her communication, I asked her what she noticed about her story in reference to her speech. The client responded that she was stuck in the belief that she would never improve. Through our discussion, the client realized that she was not acknowledging her progress. At this point, I explained that there were two choices available and that ultimately, I would accept either choice. We could continue to work together with an increased willingness on her part to journal her daily progress by using her ABCD grid (as seen later in the chapter), or we could enlist the guidance of a mental health counselor to work more specifically on her pessimistic thinking. The client decided to continue with the work we were doing, and because this was her choice, she was more likely to follow through; that is exactly what transpired.

DiLollo et al. (2003, 2005) also found that individuals who stutter do not notice their fluent periods, even after they had successfully completed treatment. They noted that, to maintain fluency, it is the clinician's responsibility to call these periods of fluency to the client's attention. These acknowledgments help clients get "unstuck" from their own self-defeating stories.

Polkinghorne (1996) classifies clients' narratives as *victimic* or *agentic*. These two types of narratives reflect the client's perceived *locus of control* (Manning, 2009; Polkinghorne, 1996), and are similar to what Seligman (2002) refers to as the *thinking styles* on the optimism–pessimism continuum. The *locus of control* refers to the degree to which a person believes that the events of her life are determined by an *external locus of control* or that the control over her life comes from external forces. An *internal locus of control* refers to the person who believes that the events in her life are largely self-determined and that the individual has control over the events in her life, or at least over how she manages these events.

The agentic narratives reflect a goal-oriented individual who takes an active role in adapting and overcoming challenges (White & Epston, 1990). Ben-Shahar (2010) referred to this role as being an *active agent* (as opposed to a passive victim) in one's life. An example of this is a PWS who views her disorder as a gift and an opportunity. This individual may view her stuttering as a chance to be more empathetic and to create a blog on the disorder and share her experiences, thoughts, and feelings with others, in being a source of comfort, strength, and inspiration to other PWS and beyond.

In contrast, *victimic narratives* indicate that the individual's view is that her life is controlled by outside forces, such as by chance and by other people. The accomplishment or failure to achieve one's life goals depends on factors that are immutable (Polkinghorne, 1996). This is when individuals function as *passive victims* in their lives (Ben-Shahar, 2010). In this type of narrative, one may hear the client say, "Look what she did to me" or "You won't believe what she did to me." A PWS may say, "I'm being punished," "Stuttering is something that happens to me," and "I've tried everything and just don't want to speak up anymore," or "The more I try to control it the worse it gets."

An example of helping a client revise her narrative is to ask the client the following questions:

- Can you describe a time when your difficulty did not get in your way of being successful?

- How do you manage to read the contractual agreements at work, given your reading difficulty?

- How did you manage to read your Spanish presentation with so much confidence? (Stacey, 1997)

These questions help our clients expand their narratives and to take on a new and adaptive perspective of themselves and of their situation. The questions aid clients in modifying their original story to a more empowering one (Wolter, DiLollo, & Apel, 2006). Just as in the SFBT approach, the clinician may ask the client with language learning disability (LLD), for example, how she has overcome her literacy challenges in the past. The more detail the client provides in her description of his abilities, the greater the chance that her new story will replace her old defeatist narrative. In this way, a narrative approach to counseling may be incorporated in a client's language and literacy intervention.

Ask Yourself

Write an example of a story one of your clients told you that reflects a victimic narrative and one that exemplifies an agentic narrative. How did you, or how could you, help the client modify her victimic narrative to one that is more agentic?

THE COGNITIVE MODEL

As mentioned previously in the Intentional Resiliency Framework (Nourse, 2015), one of the strategies for building resilience is increasing self-awareness and modifying negative thinking patterns. Aaron Beck pioneered the cognitive model in counseling and psychology in the 1960s. More recently, cognitive therapy has become a user-friendly, simple, and powerful method to help change our thoughts, build our resilience, and transform our lives. The skills of cognitive therapy, which support the development of resilience, may be successfully incorporated into the intervention we deliver as speech-language pathologists (Cook & Botterill, 2009; Menzies, Onslow, Packman, & O'Brian, 2009).

The following counseling approach is a specific way to increase resilience.

The ABCs of Flexible Thinking

Negative thoughts run through our minds all day, whether or not we're conscious of them; they're called *negative automatic thoughts* (NATs; Burns, 1999) or *automatic negative thoughts* (ANTs; Cook & Botterill, 2009). As we do the work on ourselves in this chapter, we will learn how to apply the process to our clients and families.

How do you react if someone you know walks by you and doesn't say hello? Do you have a pessimistic interpretation style? Do your NATs rant on about how that person must not care for you or is angry with you about something you did? Do your NATs prompt you to scour your memory for the moment you offended the person? If not, are you a realistic optimist who assumes that the person was engrossed in thought, did not see you, or had a recent fight with her partner and thus is distracted by something that has nothing to do with you?

What do your NATs say when your boss sends a message that she wants to speak with you? Are you immediately frozen in fear, assume that you must have done something wrong? Are your NATs telling you that you will probably get fired and never find another job? Do your NATs remind you that everything is going wrong in your life lately, so why not this? Imagine the effect that your NATs then have on your ability to think clearly, on your feelings, and ultimately on your reactions.

Ask Yourself

Write an example of a specific time when your NATs were ranting loudly. What were they saying to you?

Aaron Beck discovered links between what he called *A—adversity* (the problem), *B—beliefs* (NATs), and *C—consequences* (feelings, somatic responses, and behavioral reactions). Consider as an example of an ABC cycle, a college student we'll call Mary, who presented with a foreign accent. Her *adversity* was that she did not participate in class. Her *beliefs* were that when she contributed to class discussions, others looked at her, whispered among themselves, and thought that she had an odd way of speaking and must be unintelligent. Mary's *consequences* included anxiety, worry, nervousness, sadness, frustration, sweaty palms, shaky hands, and butterflies in her stomach. Ultimately, she continued to avoid speaking in the classroom and accumulated absences. Her grades began to fall and she then viewed herself as poor student and poor public speaker. As you can see, her behavior influenced further thoughts about her self-concept.

The Vicious Cycle

Our maladaptive patterns often begin with a thought, which drives our emotions, which drive our reactions, which affect our self-perception and ultimately our self-esteem. Once we are clear on what that initial thought was, we can get on with the business of pulling ourselves out of a maladaptive cycle.

Our goal is to notice the cycle we spin for ourselves and unravel it by identifying A, B, and C. To that list, let's add *D—disputation* (reframing or modifying the NATs into more realistic and positive thoughts). With *disputation*, we may continue to make our responses to adversity flexible and productive. In our practice of speech/language therapy, we facilitate divergent thinking in our clients (e.g., LLD, aphasia). It is important for us to apply this type of flexible thinking when any of us experience negative thoughts.

The Components of the Cycle

A tabulated grid is a useful visual tool for unraveling the cycle. The grid's columns can be labeled as follows:

- *Adversity (A)*—written in neutral terms without any emotional charge (e.g., child who does not want to read aloud because of her dyslexia).
- *Belief (B)*—may also be described in a phrase or sentence, and must be distinct from the mood or emotion (e.g., "I know I am going to make too many mistakes and read too slowly.")
- *Consequence (C)*—the mood or feeling part, which is best described in a single word (e.g., embarrassed, afraid, or nervous).
  - *Visceral or somatic responses* involve body reactions (e.g., butterflies, tightening in the stomach, feeling shaky, or trembling).
- *Disputation (D)*—refutes the *hot thought* (e.g., the thought with the greatest emotional charge) and supports reframing or modifiying this thought. For instance, the child

with dyslexia may be worried about not being able to read at all, making too many mistakes, reading too slowly, or not understanding what she read. She may also fear that the other children will make fun of her. The child selects one of these thoughts as the hot thought, which she then disputes. If she selects, "I won't be able to read at all," she may reframe that statement with, "I will read the very best I can; the teacher knows I am trying. I have never been completely unable to read in the past. Plenty of other students have reading difficulties or other problems. I'm really good at sports. The more I practice, the better I read." The more disputations generated by the client, the more effective the process.

When we dispute a thought, we look for evidence that the thought is not 100% true. One thing Robinson (2015) recommended for his students and clients is to journal about the reactions of others to their new speech or voice patterns. Journaling helps them highlight the evidence that while they may perceive themselves as sounding strange, the others' reactions prove otherwise. To gather further evidence, Robinson recommends assigning *in-therapy work* with another individual outside of the therapy room. When the other person reacts positively to the client's or student's new way of speaking, it further supports evidence for a more positive disputation.

Once you become comfortable using the vocabulary of the cycle, you're ready to play with your flexible thinking and resilience.

Ask Yourself

1. Take a look at the following mood/emotion list. Each block is one word. To further clarify feelings, fill in the bottom with additional moods you come up with on your own (adapted from Burns, 1999).

MOOD LIST					
Happy	Joyful	Excited	Stimulated	Engaged	Enthralled
Despair	Depressed	Sad	Nervous	Fearful	Anxious
Shaky	Embarrassed	Pensive	Inspired	Diminished	Frustrated

2. To be sure that you can distinguish among beliefs (thoughts), moods (emotions), and adversity (problems), take a minute to complete the following exercise. Label each of

Adversity	Belief	Consequence	Disputation
My Talk	I will forget what I will need to say	Anxious	I can check my notes
	I will not have enough time to finish the talk	Anxious	I always get done
	They will not find this useful	Anxious; down	Some may not find it useful
			All my talks have been successful
			This is a process of hard work, but works out in the end

Rating before the grid was completed:

0 _____X_____ 10

Rating after the grid was completed:

0 _____X_____ 10

Figure 8-1. ABCD grid. (Adapted from Burns, D. D. (1999). *The feeling good handbook.* New York, NY: Plume.)

the following items as an adversity, belief (thought), or consequence (mood/feeling; adapted from Burns, 1999):

a. Humiliated _____

b. Elated _____

c. I'm in big trouble _____

d. Speaking out at a work meeting _____

e. My husband's attitude _____

f. Everything is falling apart _____

g. Guilty _____

h. I'll never get the job _____

i. Comforting a grieving friend _____

j. Uneasy _____

3. Figure 8-1 is an example of my (CSR) completed ABCD grid before a presentation: A = adversity, B = beliefs or thoughts, C = consequences or feelings, D = disputation.

4. Figure 8-2 is a blank grid for practice with your own particular past or future adversity. Be sure to circle the hot thought, the one with the most emotional charge. The hot thought is the thought you will want to dispute with a more rational thought or one that is closer to true. Figure 8-3 explains how this model is relevant to stuttering.

Adversity (the problem)	Belief (NAT)	Consequence (emotion)	Disputation (evidence against)

Circle Hot Thought

Rating before the grid was completed:

0 _____ 10

Rating after the grid was completed:

0 _____ 10

Figure 8-2. Sample blank ABCD resilience grid. (Adapted from Greenberger, D., & Padesky, C. A. (1995). *Mind over mood: Change how you feel by changing the way you think*. New York, NY: Guilford Press.)

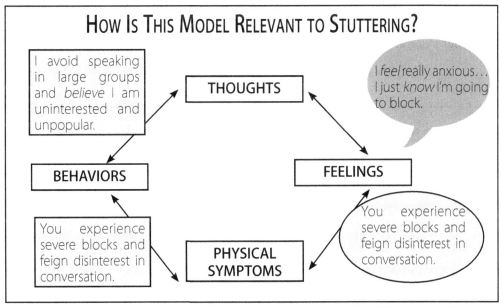

Figure 8-3. Relevance to stuttering. (Reprinted with permission from Stein-Rubin, C., & Eichorn, N. (2010). *The resilience factor: The importance of increasing resilience in individuals who stutter.* Presented at the 10th Annual National Stuttering Association Conference, Vancouver, British Columbia, Canada.)

Thinking Traps

We create our own misery by telling ourselves irrational and untrue statements. Although it is important to honor and experience negative emotions that are based in reality, when we create the negative emotions by distorting reality, we compromise our coping mechanisms. Burns (1999) described 10 thinking traps or forms of distorted thinking that lead to negative moods and interfere with our resilience. In Chapter 9, we elaborate on these traps as we discuss judgments, expectations, and the inner critic—the obstacles that interfere with and detract from the growth of ourselves as facilitators.

To summarize, we can develop more flexible and optimistic thinking styles by heightening our awareness of and challenging our NATs. In turn, we'll strengthen our resilience and self-esteem.

Ask Yourself

Answer the following questions as honestly as possible.

1. On the basis of what you now know about the characteristics of resilient individuals, what can you do to increase your resilience?

2. In which ways do your beliefs about yourself hold you back? In which ways do your beliefs about yourself contribute to your success?

3. Think of a particular situation that makes you apprehensive. Identify the adversity, reframe the NAT, and change the situation from a threat to a challenge. Become aware of your visceral changes (Ben-Shahar, 2010).

KEY CONCEPTS

- Resilience is the ability to overcome major obstacles, to steer through the trials and tribulations of everyday life, to bounce back from adversity, and to reach out of one's comfort zone.
- Reaching out is the most proactive strength.
- Resilience can be taught.
- Although as speech-language pathologists we are not psychologists, we must be adept at dealing with normal human emotions associated with a communication disorder.
- The iceberg metaphor pertains to all communication disorders and handicapping conditions in general, not only to stuttering.
- Realistic optimism is different from unrealistic optimism.
- Positive and negative interpretation styles influence how we interpret the events of our lives.
- NATs are negative automatic thoughts that become self-limiting beliefs. Beck connected adversity, thoughts, and feelings.

- Developing awareness of your ABCDs helps to make thinking styles more flexible and adaptive.

- Resigning to our NATs creates a vicious cycle of self-destructive behavior.

- The narrative model involves examining a client's personal story about her struggle. This helps the clinician gain access to the client's self-concept.

- The goal of narrative therapy is to help the client change her story to one that is more adaptive and positive.

- As we increase our resilience, we also increase self-confidence and self-esteem, improve relationships, and enhance work satisfaction.

REFERENCES

Ben-Shahar, T. (2010). *Foundations of positive psychology* [PowerPoint slides]. Retrieved from www.slideshare.net/dadalaolang/1504-01intro?ref=http://positivepsychologyprogram.com/harvard-positive-psychology-course

Burns, D. D. (1999). *The feeling good handbook*. New York, NY: Plume.

Camus, A. (1970). *Lyrical and critical essays* (E. Conroy-Kennedy, Trans.). New York, NY: Vintage Books.

Cook, F., & Botterill, W. (2009). *Tools for success: A cognitive behavioral therapy taster* [DVD]. Boston, MA: Stuttering Foundation of America.

DiLollo, A., Manning, W. H., & Neimeyer, R. A. (2003). Cognitive anxiety as a function of speaker role for fluent speakers and persons who stutter. *Journal of Fluency Disorders, 283*, 167–186.

DiLollo, A., Manning, W. H., & Neimeyer, R. A. (2005). Cognitive complexity as a function of speaker role for adult persons who stutter. *Journal of Constructivist Psychology, 183*, 215–236.

DiLollo, A., & Neimeyer, R. (2014). *Reconstructing personal narratives*. San Diego, CA: Plural Publishing.

Frankl, V. E. (1985). *Man's search for meaning*. New York, NY: Simon & Schuster.

Frid, I., Oehlen, J., & Bergbom, I. (2003). On the use of narratives in nursing research. *Journal of Advanced Nursing, 32*(3), 695–703.

Greenberger, D., & Padesky, C. A. (1995). *Mind over mood: Change how you feel by changing the way you think*. New York, NY: Guilford Press.

Kingsley, E. P. (1987). *Welcome to Holland*. Retrieved from www.child-autism-parent-cafe.com/welcome-to-holland.html

Madigan, S. P., & Goldner, E. M. (1998). A narrative approach to anorexia: Discourse, reflexivity, and questions. In M. F. Hoyt (Ed.), *The handbook of constructive therapies: Innovative approaches from leading practitioners*. San Francisco, CA: Jossey-Bass.

Manning, W. H. (2009). *Clinical decision making in fluency disorders* (3rd ed.). San Diego, CA: Singular.

Menzies, R. G., Onslow, M., Packman, A., & O'Brian, S. (2009). Cognitive behavior therapy for adults who stutter: A tutorial for speech-language pathologists. *Journal of Fluency Disorders, 34*(3), 187–200.

Neimeyer, R. A. (1995). Constructivist psychotherapies: Features, foundations, and future directions. In R. A. Neimeyer & M. J. Mahoney (Eds.), *Constructivism in psychotherapy* (pp. 11–38). Washington, DC: American Psychological Association.

Nourse, K. (2015). Get your bounce back. *The ASHA Leader, 20*(11), 30–34. doi:10.1044/leader.FTR1.20112015.30.

Polkinghorne, D. (1996). Transformative narratives: From victimic to agentic life plots. *American Journal of Occupational Therapy, 50*(4), 299–305.

Reivich, K., & Shatté, A. (2002). *The resilience factor: 7 essential skills for overcoming life's inevitable obstacles*. New York, NY: Broadway Books.

Robinson, T. L., Jr. (2015). Handle with care. *The ASHA Leader, 20*(7), 24–25. doi: 10.1044/leader.OV.20072015.24.

Seligman, M. E. (2002). *Authentic happiness: Using the new positive psychology to realize your potential for lasting fulfillment*. New York, NY: Free Press.

Sheehan, J. G. (1970). *Stuttering: Research and therapy*. New York, NY: Harper & Row.

Stacey, K. (1997). From imposition to collaboration: Generating stories of competence. In C. Smith & D. Nylund (Eds.), *Narrative therapies with children and adolescents*. New York, NY: Guilford Press.

Stein-Rubin, C., & Eichorn, N. (2010). *The resilience factor: The importance of increasing resilience in individuals who stutter*. Presented at the 10th Annual National Stuttering Association Conference, Vancouver, British Columbia, Canada.

White, M., & Epston, D. (1990). *Narrative means to narrative ends*. New York, NY: W.W. Norton.

Winslade, J., & Monk, G. (1999). *Narrative counseling in schools: Powerful and brief.* Thousand Oaks, CA: Corwin Press.

Wolter, J. A., DiLollo, A., & Apel, K. (2006). A narrative therapy approach to counseling: A model for working with adolescents and adults with language-literacy deficits. *Language Speech Hearing Services in Schools, 37*(3), 168–177. doi: 10.1044/0161-1461(2006/019).

Yaruss, J. S. (2010). Assessing quality of life in stuttering treatment outcomes research. *Journal of Fluency Disorders, 35*(3), 190–202.

RECOMMENDED WEBSITES

Positive Psychology Center: www.ppc.sas.upenn.edu

American Psychological Association, "The Road to Resilience": www.apa.org/helpcenter/road-resilience.aspx

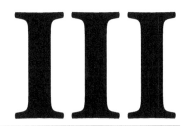

The Obstacles and Change

As we move forward in the process of transformation, we will all experience roadblocks and obstacles that will interfere with and redirect us from our goals. These obstacles will not only show up for us, they will be present for our clients and their families as well.

Judgments, disappointments, fear, anxiety, resistance, struggle, lack of confidence, guilt, and anger often influence our thinking and efforts. As human beings on the path to growth and expansion, we must learn about these obstacles that impede us. For as they throw us off our path, these obstacles may also have an impact on the people with whom we work.

Change stems from adopting powerful perspectives, developing essential skills, and addressing our obstacles. The first opportunity a clinician has to practice change, professionally, is in the clinical interview.

9

Overcoming Obstacles
Judgments, Expectations, and Inner Critic

We are all faced with a series of great opportunities brilliantly disguised as impossible situations.

—Charles Swindoll

LEARNER OUTCOMES

After reading this chapter, the reader will be able to:

1. Identify the judgments that interfere with communicating with clients and family members.

2. Recognize the attachment to expectation for clients, families, and self.

3. Describe how the inner critic interferes with the therapeutic relationship.

Up to this point, we have focused on the congruence of the clinician and the importance of empathy—acknowledging, accepting, and understanding the humanness in all of us. Furthermore, we have encouraged clinicians and facilitators to recognize that every human being, whether a client or family member, is naturally creative, resourceful, and whole—an expert on his own life circumstances. We have learned and will continue to learn to see these possibilities in others, as well as in ourselves. To expand and build on our skills as therapists and facilitators, we have focused on the importance of listening fully. We have learned that our words have an impact on whomever receives them and on the message we are trying to deliver. We have come to recognize the strengths we all possess and how to encourage the strengths in others. We have also discovered the power of resilience and the need for flexible thinking. All of these attitudes and skills guide us through the journey to transformation.

Nevertheless, the journey isn't perfect. Along the way, we inevitably exhibit behaviors that stunt our growth. We call these behaviors *the obstacles*. When we sit in judgment, when our expectations of others and ourselves are misguided, or when we relinquish

Stein-Rubin, C., & Adler, B. T. *Counseling in Communication Disorders: Facilitating the Therapeutic Rehabilitation* (pp 143-166).

power to our inner critic, we slow our movement along our path or we may veer in an undesirable direction. It is important to understand these obstacles so that we can overcome them and move forward. We present this chapter in three parts: judgments, expectations, and the inner critic.

JUDGMENTS

Real magic in relationships means an absence of judgment of others.

—Wayne Dyer

Stephen Covey (1989) relates a true story about a time when he was on a train, late at night, with several other passengers. Sitting nearby was a father and his two children, who were acting rambunctiously. The passengers were clearly annoyed and frustrated that the father wasn't quieting his children. Covey asked the father to control his children and quiet them down. The gentleman looked up, revealing a dazed expression and apologized, stating that they were coming from the hospital where his wife had just passed away and the children had not yet been informed, although he believed they were feeling it.

Although it is human nature to *judge* (to form an opinion or make a decision based on careful thought), the operative words here are *careful thought*. How often are we careful about our judgments, and how quickly do we make them? Julia Cameron (2002) suggested that it is wise not to judge too quickly or too early. Nevertheless, we quickly judge others by their appearance, on what they say, on their actions, and on their choices. We may judge people on whether they strike us as compatible with who we are, with how we look, and with what we say and do.

If we accept that making judgments is human and to be expected, then why is there a problem? The problem with judging is what we *do* with our judgment. We must be aware of the extent to which we let our opinions influence how we treat others. Judging may often obstruct our view of another person. Even when we think we're listening, our unconscious judgments may dictate what we hear and the actions we take toward someone else. We do not want our judgments to shut down the effectiveness of our communication and interfere with our goal of empowering therapeutic relationships. This awareness is as important in our personal lives as it is in our professional ones.

In the clinical realm, our student clinicians meet individuals from many cultures and backgrounds. They are often faced with children who may be the products of divorce, living with parents of same-sex marriages, individuals who wear traditional clothing from their culture, or those who have different socioeconomic backgrounds and native languages. There may be differences related to vocal tone and projection as well as mannerisms. Student clinicians have shared that they have difficulty controlling their snap judgments about these individuals. As clinicians and facilitators, we must recognize our tendencies to judge others for their differences and acknowledge how our judgments may interfere with our communication, interactions, and perspective. Refer to the American Speech-Language-Hearing Association website about cultural difference (www.asha.org/slp/CLDinSchools). Fill out and review the American Speech-Language-Hearing Association (ASHA) Cultural Competence Checklist in Appendix A in order to better understand yourself in relation to others who are culturally different.

As we learn about our judgments, we must be willing to acknowledge and notice that other people are most likely judging us in a variety of ways and for different reasons. We may all face moments when we feel that we are being criticized or not accepted for who we are. Richard Carlson (1997) has stated that, for some of us, to be judged is synonymous with being criticized. For example, children and teens may feel criticized and bullied by others, parents may feel criticized by teachers and clinicians, children may feel criticized by their parents, employees may feel criticized by their bosses, and clients may feel criticized by the clinicians. When individuals perceive these comments as judgments and criticisms, they tend to shut down and retreat (Faber & Mazlish, 2012). The deliverer of the feedback then feels judged and rejected, so he in turn shuts down and retreats. These perceptions and behaviors create a vicious cycle, which precludes effective communication.

Another type of judgment occurs with self-judgment. Sometimes these judgments are too harsh and influence our behaviors, causing us to retreat as described. We may experience a loss of confidence. If self-judgment goes too far, the inner critic takes over. We will discuss the inner critic in depth later in this chapter.

The impact of judgments is extensive. Judgments may encourage and discourage us. They may propel us forward or stop us in our tracks. We must be aware of the ones we make and learn how to deal with the ones made of us to assist our clients and their families in the therapeutic process and to improve our communication in the therapeutic relationship.

Judgment Versus Evaluation

Because we have acknowledged that all human beings judge, it's also important to distinguish judgment from evaluation. According to Haynes and Pindzola (2011), the word *evaluative* denotes objectivity, whereas *judgment* implies subjectivity. Evaluation allows for spaciousness and possibility; when we adopt an evaluative stance, we are not sure exactly how things will turn out—we're exploring. In contrast, judgment implies finality, restriction, and a premeditated decision. Judgments may be off-putting and uncomfortable. Even unspoken judgments, such as obvious facial expressions or body language, may compromise our effectiveness as communicators.

Ask Yourself

Let's examine and learn about our judgments as follows:

1. List two ways that you judge yourself.

2. List two ways that you judge others.

3. Write about a time when you shut down and retreated as a result of someone's judgment of you.

4. Describe how your judgments of others may affect your relationships.

Ways to Counter Judgments

The following are several effective ways to counter our judgments:

- Develop curiosity about the origin of our judgments.
- Develop curiosity about the judgments of others.
- Self-manage our reactions.
- Engage in neurolinguistic programing (NLP).

Curiosity About the Origin of Our Judgments

Curiosity is the most effective antidote to judgment (Ben-Shahar, 2010). First, we must be curious about ourselves and determine where our judgments come from; that list will likely include our family of origin, friends, culture, traditions, and religion. Understanding where our judgments stem from may help us forgive ourselves for being judgmental. Through self-awareness, we will find ways to shift, alter, and manage our thoughts and observations.

Part of becoming self-aware means noticing our reactions to judgments. For example, when a parent of a client questions our methods, we may feel criticized (e.g., "He must not see me as competent" or "She thinks I don't know what I'm talking about"). At the same time, we may feel critical of the parent for questioning us. This response is often the defense that may surface when we interpret a judgment as criticism. We may then try to appear all-knowing, providing every possible rationale for our choices to ensure full, judgment-free acceptance. Here is where we need curiosity. The questions that we could ask ourselves are the following: Is it possible that the parent is defensive to avoid our judgment? Is it possible that we become defensive to avoid being perceived as wrong (Box 9-1)?

Box 9-1
A speech-language pathologist relayed a story about a time when a mother entered the room for her son's first session and was exasperated that therapy had been scheduled at an inconvenient time of day. She adamantly expressed her frustration to the clinician who, instead of understanding and acknowledging the mother's dilemma, responded that *(continued)*

Box 9-1 (CONTINUED)
there were no other time slots available. Their interaction became tense and adversarial until finally the clinician brought the child in and began the session. Afterward, the clinician felt regretful about her mismanagement of the situation. She realized that her judgments reflected her own frustrations related to managing her own time and meeting her own responsibilities. Her judgments of the mother interfered with establishing a collaborative partnership and trust.

Curiosity About the Judgments of Others

Because the antidote to judgment is curiosity (Kimsey-House, Kimsey-House, Sandahl, & Whitworth, 2011), we must maintain a curious stance with our clients and their families. As we explore our discomfort when the person sitting across from us is tearful or frustrated, we must consider that a parent's reactions may stem from an underlying cause such as grief, sadness, or anger in response to a catastrophic change (Luterman, 2008).

When we learn to listen at a deep level, we hear parents judge themselves, express their fear of outside judgment, and mourn the loss of a dream. As clinicians, when we judge family members, we may overlook the family's struggle with the difficult news they've received. We have observed and overheard our student clinicians judging a family's responses without realizing that the family's reactions may be normal coping mechanisms in times of loss. The following are several of the worries, fears, and losses that parents have acknowledged in our therapy room:

- The dream of a normal and perfect child, who meets their personal standards (Kingsley, 1987).
- The dream of protecting that child from harm regardless of the circumstances.
- The dream of who they are in the world as defined by their roles, which no longer fit or apply.
- Mothers of children with special needs often blame themselves for some failure during pregnancy or during parenting (Luterman, 2008).
- Parents may blame themselves for their secret negative feelings about their lot in life.
- Fathers often blame themselves if the security and comfort of the family is challenged. If the burden of the special need is financial, the father frequently carries that stress (Luterman, 2008).

Although the client may not be emotionally ready, the clinician may find himself anxious for a client to move on to acceptance and then judge him for not moving forward. As we learn to make a space for our clients' grief, we must not impose a time limit. We suggest the following:

- Avoid judging other people's grieving processes
- Access your compassion and understanding, listening abilities, and willingness to provide the support that may be needed

On the other hand, if the grief has gone on for extended periods of time and is interfering with the individual's functioning, it may be necessary to make a referral to a mental health counselor.

Self-Management of Our Reactions

Self-management is the ability to control one's emotions in reaction to a client or a client's story. Self-management is critical to our discussion on judgment. Certain stories, events, or examples that a client relates about his life may touch a chord in us and cause us to react. If we, as clinicians, give in to this subjective tug, we run the risk of clouding our objectivity and of allowing the focus of the client to fall. It is one thing to share self when the time is right; it is another thing to get pulled into an emotional spiral that could interfere with our evaluation of the client's or family's situation.

An example of self-management would be if a client, in a clinical interview, relates information about his divorce and you have been divorced; this could evoke your empathy. Nevertheless, you would need to self-manage your emotions to be fully present for the client.

Another example of the need to self-manage is when a client may remind you of someone whom you dislike. Our facial expression and body language could reveal our feelings (Flasher & Fogle, 2012). There could be a strong need to self-manage here to get to a place where we may be fully neutral and present for the client (Whitworth, 2007).

When we evaluate children or adults, we must self-manage our reactions according to the client's or family member's temperament. Understanding the client's temperament helps guide the clinician in terms of his attitude, reactions, and responses (Carey & McDevitt, 1995; Riley, 2002). Knowing this contributes to the success of connecting with the client while working within his framework of tolerance (Griffith & Frieden, 2000).

When assessing difficult-to-test children, remember that there are always options. For example, when working with a 3-year-old child who enters the evaluation room tearful and clinging to his mother, it may be necessary to modify the original plans for the evaluation. First, invite the parent to join the clinician on the floor using a few select toys. If the child resists your requests to engage in floor play or displays signs of anxiety, avoid excessive requesting and questioning. Manolson, Ward, and Dodington (1995) used the acronym AAA to clarify how to engage with a child in play. AAA means the following:

- *Allow* the child to lead.
- *Adapt* to share the moment.
- *Add* new experiences and words.

If the child refuses to respond to the clinician, the clinician may remove himself from the immediate area, view the child from a distance, and prompt the parent accordingly.

Ask Yourself

1. How many times do you think a clinician has criticized parental behavior before attempting to get curious, deeply listen, assist, guide, and support? How often have you engaged in that kind of judgment?

2. How frequently do we reflexively shift into judgment mode when parents do not follow our recommendations? Provide an example.

3. We can say from experience that when parents or new clinicians do not do as they have been told, we may judge them negatively. We suggest getting curious about the parents' actions. Describe a time when you have gotten curious about a parent's behavior rather than judging him.

Neurolinguistic Programming

We believe that a key to dissolving judgment is in the saying, "Before you judge another, walk a mile in his shoes." The question is, how do we get to that place where we are actually in the other person's shoes without being the other person? A useful approach to help answer this question is in NLP. NLP is an approach to communication and psychotherapy created by Richard Bandler and John Grinder in California in the 1970s. Bandler and Grinder noticed connections among the neurological processes (*neuro*), language (*linguistic*), and behavioral patterns learned through experience (*programming*). These components may be changed to achieve specific goals. By using the four NLP personas, or perceptual positions (as described next, we may create a sense of another person's experience through our imaginations, memories, and other senses. When we engage in this role play, it is important to have the client move to another location, such as another chair or sitting vs standing (Hoag, 2015).

In the *First Position*, or perspective, we imagine everything, whether past or future, as if it is happening in the present. For example, if we were picturing a time when we were children, we would imagine these events as if they were happening right now.

The *Second Position* is the *other* position. *Other* may refer to people as another perspective. In this position, we get into character, and try to embody the thoughts and feelings of *other*. The unique part of this exercise is that the Second Position may be in verbal communication with the First Position. When talking to Second Position from First, or from First Position to Second, use the pronoun "you" to make the conversation genuine.

The *Third Position* is that of the curious observer. As the observer, we are not a part of the dialogue between First and Second Positions; however, we are there to observe the dialogue, including the dynamics in the relationship. In Third Position, use the third-person pronoun, "he" or "she" to refer to oneself.

In the *Fourth Position*, we are able to see the fusion of the other three systems and feel the integration of the whole. Tendencies and patterns become clarified from this perspective.

When a clinician is faced with a genuine or imagined conflict, NLP may provide a facilitating tool. For example, a clinician may feel frustrated when interacting with his clinical supervisor who may have some valid points that she has been trying to express to the clinician. Nevertheless, the clinician is consumed with his point of view and judgments, just as the supervisor is judging the clinician. This cycle of judgment causes significant anxiety and strain on the relationship and on their communication. In this case, the student-clinician may engage in an NLP role-play where he plays the part of himself (First Position) and of his supervisor (Second Position). This dialogue may facilitate the clinician's understanding of the supervisor's reaction thereby leading to a more realistic and adaptive reaction.

Clinically, NLP could work effectively for a speech-language pathologist's client who may be a person who stutters (PWS). In this case, the PWS is self-conscious about speaking up in class, assuming that another student is staring at him because of his speech. The speech-language pathologist may employ the NLP approach to assist the PWS to assess the point of view of his fellow student more adaptively. While assuming the role of his fellow student, the PWS may discover that his classmate was in fact looking at him to pay attention, that she may have difficulty focusing, or that she admired the PWS's ideas and courage to speak up in class.

If we learn to quiet the voices of judgment by maintaining an open curious attitude toward others and ourselves, focus on self-management, and incorporate the four positions that NLP describes, we have greater control of judgments. Learning about judgments and how to counter them helps us find common ground, open up communication, and facilitate powerful therapeutic relationships.

EXPECTATIONS

When you stop expecting people to be perfect, you can like them for who they are.
—Donald Miller, 2011

Expectation refers to a strong belief that something will happen or be the case in the future. It is not unreasonable for us as human beings to expect the best of others, ourselves, and our life situations. In our field, supervisors and instructors expect to have students who fulfill their assignments and students often expect to have instructors and supervisors who are warm, encouraging, and supportive. As speech-language pathologists, audiologists, clinicians, and facilitators, we expect to be knowledgeable, effective, and engaging with our clients. From discussions with the families we work with we know that parents usually expect to have normal and healthy children that will develop within expectancy, conform to the rules, and succeed in school. In the big picture, our expectations may foster our growth and serve to motivate our achievement, particularly, if they are realistic and achievable.

On the other hand, there is a downside to expectations. We have all experienced disappointments in our lives. When we look closely, we realize that most disappointments were the result of unfulfilled expectations. As a result we may make comments such as, "I try never to expect anything," or "My expectations always lead to disappointment," or "People always disappoint me. That's why I have no close friends." Sometimes we shut down, avoid trying again, or just give up.

The reality is that expectations that are low diminish a person's performance and expectations that are held high may encourage and increase performance (Buckingham & Clifton, 2001). Yet if expectations are unrealistic and stem from perfectionism, they may create frustration and disappointment. If they are realistic and achievable, they can be motivating and expanded upon. We also learned that it is important to state our expectations clearly and respectfully in professional and personal relationships (Faber & Mazlish, 2005).

The Impact of Low Expectations

When we treat an individual as incapable, it diminishes his ability and confidence to meet his potential. When we treat a child with a particular disability by the limits described by the label, we diminish that child's potential and may actually restrict the child from progressing. When parents categorize their children, those children may live out that label for the rest of their lives. We have all heard about the personality traits of first, middle, and youngest children. Although sometimes we fit some of these traits, we would not want to be limited by them or to have the label define who we are (Sapey & Oliver, 2006). For example, when one child is known as the "pretty one" and her sibling is known as the "smart one," this point of view may diminish the pretty one's motivation to live out her potential as an intelligent human being (Boxes 9-2 and 9-3). The smart one may resign to slow self-esteem regarding her appearance. As noted in Chapter 3, labels may lead to negative self-fulfilling prophecies.

Box 9-2

In 1951, my (BTA) second brother was born with Down's syndrome. My parents were young; my mother was 26, and my father was 29. I was 6, and my other brother was 18 months old. We didn't know what was going on. My parents talked all the time about my new brother's appearance. The doctors were not helpful and said they couldn't explain the nature of this to my mother and father, that my brother was unusual. My mother withdrew and my father began making inquiries. I thought he was adorable with blond hair and blue eyes. He was happy and affectionate.

My parents took him to a major hospital specializing in children who are different and with disabilities. They were told that he was "mongoloid," would never learn, would live a totally unproductive life, and that my parents must consider putting my brother in an institution. These were the days of Willowbrook Institution. That was all they needed to hear, and everyone swung into action. There was no way that this child would be institutionalized.

Early Intervention did not exist at that time. My mother became the therapist, observing, supporting, and teaching all that she could. We loved him so much and he loved us. He learned, maybe at a slower pace and a little later, to stand up and turn over regardless of the braces on his legs. He walked and ran with us, learned how to swim, eventually to improve his speech with a therapist, and we, as a family, attended every event through AHRC and ACRMD. My brother was a model who did not meet the low expectations of the doctors. He went to Brooklyn College's Early Childhood Center for preschool and became an inspiration for teachers and psychologists who observed the children there.

(continued)

Box 9-2 (CONTINUED)

He attended school, graduated from special education classes, worked in a special educational workshop, and learned how to travel on buses. My brother loved to bowl, go to the library, and to dance. He was a loving person and had a great sense of humor. He was always a wonderful brother, brother-in-law, and uncle, and he lived to become a great uncle.

When he passed away at 63 years old, we found out how many people he served to inspire to become the teachers and doctors that they are today. Low expectations were not acceptable in our family. He was never pushed beyond; he was self-motivated and encouraged, and we truly loved him.

Box 9-3

Susan Boyle was a contestant on the TV show *Britain's Got Talent*. Her life story is a testament to strength, resilience, self-esteem, judgments, and expectations. Susan was diagnosed with Asperger's syndrome as an adult. Yet as a child, she was sorely misunderstood. At school, kids teased and mistreated her, and teachers had unrealistically low expectations of her. She did not understand herself and why she was treated the way she was.

Susan loved music and longed to be a singer. She may have had unrealistic expectations for herself, despite the fact that people constantly challenged her self-esteem. When *Britain's Got Talent* discovered Susan and her gift, they shared her beautiful voice with the world. Although her singing captivated people, they were simultaneously curious about her unusual affect. This became difficult for Susan to deal with as she attempted to be responsive to the accolades and interviews.

After her diagnosis, Susan's struggles changed. Today, Susan understands herself better than she did when she was a child, and she realizes why she might have seemed strange or different to her peers. Her battles with self-esteem, the unrealistically low expectations of others, and possibly her own unrealistic expectations to be a singer were countered by her inner strength and resilience. Her love of music and singing were so strong that she maintained a determination do what she loved. With the support of *Britain's Got Talent*, she made a name for herself as a singer and now speaks publicly about her Asperger's. She says that her life has improved. Perhaps that's because Susan is no longer the object of judgments or the expectations of others.

The Impact of Realistically High Expectations

When we hold high expectations, there is an increase in performance (Buckingham & Clifton, 2001). We want to encourage our students and clients to meet their goals. We want our clients to succeed in school and know they can achieve the grades they need to move on to college, if that is what they choose. In any job we hold, we are expected to meet the standards of the position with focus and determination to succeed. This is not necessarily because our employer is trying to be difficult; it may simply be a job requirement. When we meet this requirement, we may be proud of ourselves for fulfilling that expectation. This is how we learn and grow. Those of us who are health conscious may have high expectations related to exercise and diet to maintain good health as we age. Weekly articles in the *New York Times* Science section speak to this issue (e.g., Brody, 2015). All of these are *realistic expectations*, which are achievable and within reason—goals we set that won't lead to frustrations. They are reachable if one works toward them step by step. Therefore, having realistically high expectations and the willingness to step out of the box may build resilience and self-esteem.

Unrealistically High Expectations

Sometimes whether an expectation is realistic or not depends on the situation and person; what's realistic for you may not be realistic for someone else and vice versa. Therefore, a common problem many of us face is that some of our expectations may be held unrealistically high. Unrealistic expectations are usually unachievable and frustrating goals. For example, it is unrealistic to expect yourself or anyone else to be a fully skilled doctor or clinician without the necessary years of training and experience. It may be financially unrealistic to purchase a particular house without adequate funds or to expect an individual with a disability to overcome the struggle with just a few visits to a specialist. It is unrealistic for us to expect a spouse, partner, and good friend to be able to read our minds and know what we want so that our expectation of them may be fulfilled.

When it comes to personal and professional success, we often unrealistically place too much demand on others and ourselves to recognize our accomplishments (Cameron, 2002). When parents overdo recognition of success or overdo praise for their children's efforts through the years, the adult children come to expect recognition from others. Research about the Millenial generation and *helicopter parents* (parents who hover over their children) has reported that students who have been praised extensively by their parents will often drop out of classes because they are fearful of receiving a less-than-perfect grade. Some are afraid of even choosing a major.

In our practices, we have students who say that the only acceptable grade is an A, and if they get a B, they feel that they have failed. As a result of excessive build up and praise, we may see parents coming to teachers at all levels of education, including college campuses, to speak for their adult children about weak grades. They believe that the weaker grades will lower their child's self-esteem. As children move on in school, teachers and instructors are usually more concerned with a child performing to his potential, not just feeling good. Bronson and Merryman (2009) relate that young adults today tend to be immature. We have heard stories about parents who call their adult child's boss to complain that their adult child did not receive a bonus.

In our field, it is unrealistic for a supervisor to expect a new student-clinician to have the same level of skill that the supervisor has spent years learning. This has been a frequent frustration and complaint of many new clinicians. At the same time, it is often difficult for new student-clinicians to set realistic and achievable goals for their clients. Sometimes the steps our student-clinicians choose are far too complex to be accomplished. The client may then become frustrated with therapy when he cannot achieve the goals. We have observed clinicians request that children with literacy problems read books that they are unable to master, particularly if they have not accomplished the earlier levels with success.

Both personally and professionally, we may expect a great deal from other people, while at the same time, these individuals may have impossibly high expectations of us. We may learn during a parent conference that we are not fulfilling a parent's expectations. Just as we may learn that we are also not fulfilling the expectations of someone else in our lives. During the Therapeutic Relationship course at Brooklyn College in New York, our students have freely expressed their frustrations related to their own personal and professional expectations of others. At the same time, students do not like to be on the receiving end of someone else's expectations of them. They may perceive these expectations as unfair and unreasonable. When this dichotomy occurs, both individuals become defensive and angry; these emotions may then thwart their communication and diminish the relationship. These unrealistically high expectations create a vicious cycle of unfulfilled expectations and a negative self-fulfilling prophecy.

Ask Yourself

Let us identify our expectations on several levels.

1. List two personal or professional expectations that are achievable (realistic).

2. List two personal or professional expectations that are unrealistic.

3. List two expectations that you have of others. Are they realistic? Would the other person perceive them as realistic?

4. List two expectations that others have of you and state whether you perceive them as realistic or unrealistic.

Disappointments Have a History

When we are disappointed, our reaction to the present event may often be compounded by similar experiences from the past. This phenomenon has been called a *stack attack* and can be powerful. For example, the woman who becomes disappointed with a friendship overreacts to a small incident with a friend. Upon examining her history, one finds that she has had several failed friendships in which another person has disappointed her. As a result, she may isolate herself and decide to remain friendless. Children who are abandoned by a parent may have trust issues later in life. A PWS may go through a single situation where they have a severe block during a presentation. The PWS might overgeneralize that this will then occur in all of his presentations. We may sabotage relationships and/or new situations unless we work on our awareness of the source for these reactions. We must maintain awareness of our reactions and of their source so that we do not end up sabotaging our relationships.

When our personal and professional expectations, both the realistic and the unrealistic ones, are thwarted, our disappointments may color our judgments and attitudes and affect our communication skills. How we handle disappointments says a great deal about who we are, and about how effective we will be as counselors. It is worthwhile, in the big picture, to develop a sense of humor about the unrealistic expectations we set for ourselves and the unrealistic expectations that others set for us. After all, it's rather humorous how often we try to achieve what is not humanly possible.

Ask Yourself

1. Think about an expectation you had that went unfulfilled. How intense was your disappointment? What did the feeling remind you of from the past (history stack attack)?

2. Think about an expectation someone had for you that you didn't fulfill. How did you experience that person's disappointment? How did your feelings influence how you listened, spoke to, and related to that person?

THE INNER CRITIC

There once was a cruel goblin who had an evil idea. He crafted a mirror that could reflect only flaws. One day, the evil goblin decided he would take the mirror up to heaven, so that the angels would see themselves in this ugly way. On the way up to heaven, the goblin dropped the mirror, and it smashed into countless pieces. Each shard settled into all of the people's eyes and hearts. The people only saw and felt what was ugly or flawed about them. The evil goblin laughed and laughed.

(Adapted from "The Snow Queen" by Hans Christian Andersen 1844/1983)

We all possess an *inner critic* or *inner critical voice*. We experience this voice as a negative internal commentary on who we are and how we behave (Firestone, Firestone, & Catlett, 2002). Sometimes we see ourselves as ugly and unlovable, and our inner critics or saboteurs[1] may keep us from reaching our full potential (Kimsey-House et al., 2011). People vary in their approaches to coping with this aspect of the self. How we relate to our inner critic profoundly influences how we perceive, react to, and relate to situations and to other people, as well as how we rally from adversity.

---

[1] Please note that the words *inner critic* and *saboteur* will be used interchangeably throughout this section.

The inner critic develops when we are young as an outgrowth of the warnings of parents, grandparents, siblings, and teachers. To keep us safe, our elders tell us over and over, "Be careful," "Don't hurt yourself," "Be realistic," and so on, and these messages become embedded in our consciousness. As we grow, those internalized warnings caution us to stay safe by staying in our comfort zone. And we do stay safe; sometimes too safe, because the inner critic scares us and makes us doubt our own abilities. After all, we can handle a little discomfort, can't we? In fact, without discomfort, we do not grow (Ben-Shahar, 2010).

The critic's voice, combined with current internal and external (often unrealistic) demands, can make us believe we are inadequate, incompetent, inferior, undeserving, unworthy, or powerless. This saboteur may also emerge under the guise of confusion, fear, anxiety, lack of clarity, or emptiness. It will tell you, "You are not thin enough, attractive enough, accomplished enough, smart enough, capable enough; you are not *enough*. You are not a good enough partner, parent, or grandparent. You will never make it; this is not realistic; you are defective, broken, worthless, and inappropriate. You are not a fully developed person like other people." Sound familiar?

It is important to note that the critic doesn't want us to strive for personal growth. He is threatened anytime we attempt to change the status quo by taking a life-enhancing risk. Heifetz, Grashow, and Linsky (2009) talk about using discomfort to drive progress rather than repressing it to restore the comfortable status quo. Ideally, we may take risks anyway; however, the more we accomplish, the more the critic goes into a tailspin. As a result, we second-guess our own decisions, which may lead us to indecisiveness and procrastination. In fact, it is our continuous improvement that ought to be the norm, and the status quo is what we need to question (Cawsey & Descza, 2011).

The inner critic is therefore a product and manifestation of expectations imposed on us early in our lives. However, the impact of the critic is not only a result of the elders' comments in our childhood; the critic's voice gathers strength from all kinds of negative experiences and relationships such as bullying, friendships gone wrong, or any variation of the norm including a speech-language, hearing, or learning disorder.

The Inner Critic and Self-Fulfilling Prophecy

Over time, our negative self-images may become self-fulfilling prophecies that manifest in our personal and professional lives. The critical voice is potentially so debilitating that it keeps a person from achieving. When we can't achieve, we may feel unworthy and useless, we may then act as if we are unworthy and useless, and so the vicious cycle continues. The truth is that we are not unworthy and useless; rather, we're beaten down from years of hearing about our inadequacy (Stone & Stone, 1993).

Our formed reality and core beliefs about ourselves result from the critic's internalization of our relationships, personal experiences, and the way in which we have been raised. As noted in Chapter 2, we grow uncomfortable if there is inconsistency between our core beliefs or our deep-seated view of ourselves, and what actually happens in our lives. If a person's success exceeds his poor perception of himself, he will likely self-sabotage at some point (Box 9-4).

Box 9-4

My (CSR) friend believed she was unworthy of a recent promotion. Rather than adjust her self-perception to fit this evidence of how she was valued, she rejected the position and sabotaged her efforts on the job. She began to arrive late at her workplace, made careless errors, and missed meetings to align with her saboteur, rather than believe in her true nature, her real self, who wanted to be happy. My friend's conflict must have been so great that she would have done anything to reduce her feeling of turmoil—anything to soothe herself back into her belief that she was undeserving. Once she lost the job, my friend's anxiety dissipated.

Success is just too uncomfortable for some people who believe that they're destined to fail (Ben-Shahar, 2010; Branden, 1995; Box 9-5).

Box 9-5

A clinician related a story about a high school student who stuttered. He explained that he recently met a pretty girl who was interested in his music and in spending time together. They went out on several occasions. In therapy, the boy expressed his anxiety and struggle with the idea that such a pretty girl and nice person could actually like him. Rather than allow the relationship to unfold, he constantly called and texted her. He too set himself up for a failed relationship and sabotaged his opportunity

---

Awareness and Acceptance

Because we all have an inner critic who never goes away completely, we must gain active awareness and acceptance of its subliminal voice. The inner critic can be confusing. It may slyly seem to act in our best interest; unfortunately, our best interest is the last thing this voice wants to serve. Sometimes we think this voice is the real us, when in fact, it's just trying to compete with our true inner voice. Our goal is to learn to distinguish between these two voices and remember that *we* are not our saboteur—that in fact, we have the power to observe and interact productively with the saboteur. The more conscious we are of the critic, the more empowered we are to be our true selves. We may ask ourselves, "Who is doing the talking now?" Our awareness will allow us to gently acknowledge the critic, stand strong in what we know to be true, and gently move that damaging voice aside. Only then may we become who we really are.

One of the strategies for working with the critic that Sidra and Hal Stone (1993) suggested is to journal. Speech-language pathologists may advise their clients as well as the clients' teachers to use this method as follows: The student writes out a conversation with his inner critic as though he is carrying on a dialogue with another person. They suggest a simple process: "You sit down in front of a notebook and begin to write from the 'I' that is talking to your inner critic."

Recognizing the inner critical voice in children could be helpful for classroom teachers. Box 9-6 is an example of how a math teacher created a dialogue in his classroom. This type of dialogue is also applicable for speech-language pathologists and supervisors in the clinical setting. Any one of us may find a time in our lives when this strategy may work for us both personally and professionally.

Box 9-6

In a math class, for example, after explaining the concept of the inner critic, the instructor invited the students to write a conversation between themselves and their inner math critic. The intention was to raise the students' awareness of this critical voice as being separate from who they really are and what they are capable of. What the authors refer to as a *Voice Dialogue* would look like this:

I: I want to talk to you because I'm realizing just how powerful you are and how much I listen to you.

Critic: Well, I'm glad you realize just how important I am. If you would always do what I say, like dropping this math class, I think things would go much better for you.

I: No, that isn't what I meant exactly. I appreciate your power, but I'm also becoming aware of how much you've been criticizing me all my life, especially when it comes to math.

Critic: Well, better me than the teacher. I'm just trying to keep you from being embarrassed.

I: Why do you think I will be embarrassed?

Critic: Because I know you can't do math. You have always gotten bad grades in the past.

I: That may be true, but in the past I didn't really take my math classes seriously. Now I plan to spend 2 hours every evening completing the homework and I'll ask the instructor questions if there's something I don't understand.

Critic: What makes you think you're going to change and take math seriously now?

I: Now I realize that doing well in math is a step toward my goal of becoming an engineer. (Stone & Stone, 1989)

Using the Critic to Our Advantage

Instead of relinquishing our power to the critic, we may learn to use it to our advantage. No one enjoys being criticized, especially those who have low self-esteem or perfectionistic natures; we would all rather hear positive feedback. On the other hand, criticism may be educational; we have the capacity to learn from it and to transform as a result. It's beneficial to take criticism openly and curiously, to keep what's useful and disregard the rest.

Although negative self-perception may be a strong motivator, when it is carried to extremes, it may be destructive and block happiness. In response to the inner critic, we may excel, and yet some of us are never satisfied. The curse of high achievers is climbing the perpetual mountain only to arrive at the top to see a new mountain to climb; this has been called the *perfectionistic treadmill*. Workaholics and perfectionists, who persist just to prove themselves to the critic, who is never satisfied, are left repeatedly empty and unhappy (Ben-Shahar, 2010).

Being Ourselves

If we do not learn how to be in harmony with ourselves, how will we deal with the denial, resistance, and hostility of our clients? Have you noticed any clients or family members who stand and walk tensely, who are bent or stooped, who scowl and hold tension in the jaw? Casting their eyes downward, they radiate their conviction that they do not deserve to take up space. These individuals may be in an internal battle with their critic or struggling to be "right" about their core beliefs. They may prefer to stand small rather than to risk provoking jealousy. They are their "own worst enemies" (Branden, 1995).

The inner critic keeps reminding us to stay small, to blend in, and to be inconspicuous or even invisible. It reminds us that we are undeserving. Ian Wallace's question strikes a chord when he asks, "Why are you trying so hard to fit in when you were born to stand out?" Many of us spend a great deal of our time worrying, at various levels of consciousness, about what others will think. We are so fearful of "making fools of ourselves" that we never get to be ourselves.

Ask Yourself

1. What is your shard—that negative lens through which you view yourself? (See the Andersen story about the goblin at the beginning of this section.)

   ○ Take a few moments to access your own saboteur.

   ○ What does the voice say?

   ○ What physical sensations take hold when your saboteur kicks in, and where do you feel those sensations in your body?

   ○ Is your saboteur male, female, androgynous, or a whole committee?

   ○ What situations trigger the saboteur's arrival?

○ Who in your life does your critic mirror?

2. List the phrases that the critic repeats in your head (e.g., "You're so careless," "You're so lazy," "You're too heavy"; adapted from Stone & Stone, 1993)

When we interview and counsel clients and their families, we'll often hear the other person's inner critic talking to us. We offer the example of a client's mother's comments in Box 9-7. Pay attention to her self-sabotaging voice, and then to the responses that we, the diagnosticians, may make.

Box 9-7

Client: My son will not be able to go to college. He will have to take a menial job. His skills are not good enough to become a professional. How will he ever make a living and support a family?*

Diagnostician (sample questions):

- How is this belief serving you?
- What is the benefit of believing this? What is the cost?
- What is another possibility? What is another perspective?
- Is this your opinion?
- May I offer a suggestion? Let's stay present in the now and build on the progress over time.
- I hear how much you love your son and want to protect him. What other ways are you able to show your love and support for him in this situation?
- What are your son's most important goals (e.g., after graduation, completion of this program)? How can you support these?

*It is important to note that the saboteur may rear its head at the initial meeting and become more fully expressed during the therapy process. It is the diagnostician's role to note the presence of the self-sabotaging voice and to alert the therapist who will conduct the therapy.

In terms of supervisor and student-clinician communication, a supervisor's constructive feedback may resonate with the student's inner critic. If the student has a core belief based on his critic of not being skilled enough, this may have an impact on his reactions, and his responses may then come across as defensive. For example, a student-clinician may be working with a child who exhibits delays in language development. The child surprises everyone and expresses himself in single-word utterances during the therapy session. The supervisor suggests during the course of the session that the clinician expand on the child's single-word utterances. The clinician's saboteur emphatically reprimands him, telling him that he cannot do anything right, that he should have known what to do on the spot, that he has made an unfavorable impression on his supervisor, and will probably get a poor grade. Because of those internal reactions, the clinician becomes defensive and shuts down. This impacts his relationship with the supervisor who senses the student's attitude. It's the attitude that makes a stronger impression than the fact that the student did not take the therapy to the next level. We are not expected to know what we don't know; we are expected to self-manage our attitudes.

The Inner Critic and Thinking Traps

Another way the inner critic may manifest is in the form of thinking traps (Burns, 1999; Reivich & Shatté, 2002). When we fall into a thinking trap, we become entangled in a behavior that doesn't serve us well. We have chosen five thinking traps to explore here:

1. Jumping to conclusions (catastrophizing)
   a. Mind-reading
   b. Fortune-telling
2. Overgeneralization: a form of all-or-nothing thinking
3. Personalizing and blame
4. Emotional reasoning
5. Discounting the positive

Jumping to Conclusions (Catastrophizing)

Maria speaks English as a second language. When she was chatting with a group of English-speaking peers on her college campus, she hesitated to express her thoughts. She had some definite ideas, but she held back because of her thinking traps: "They will laugh when I try to speak. They'll think I'm stupid" (mind-reading). "They won't value my opinion anyway" (fortune-telling).

Maria was jumping to conclusions—assuming without actually knowing the truth. As a result, she shut down and closed herself off from communicating with the group. That is, Maria's behavioral reaction reinforced her belief that she could not socialize with native English speakers. Her self-esteem and her feelings of fear, shame, and embarrassment were reinforced. She felt awkward and useless. She became a passive victim to her thinking trap.

Overgeneralization: A Form of All-or-Nothing Thinking

When something negative happens (e.g., romantic rejection), we may overgeneralize: "Everyone always rejects me; no one ever wants to be with me." As another example, making a mistake might lead to the self-sabotaging thought, "I always mess up."

Personalization and Blame

Personalization means taking something personally even though it's not about us, which then prevents us from getting to the root of a problem and solving it. For example, when Alice's husband was in a bad mood because he was having trouble at work, she immediately assumed she was the problem. She therefore believed she was responsible for her husband's moodiness. Rather than talking to him and listening to his feelings about whatever was bothering him, which had nothing to do with her, she blamed herself for his attitude. Alice took his mood personally and then rejected him out of this thought.

Blame, the opposite of personalization, refers to blaming others in circumstances that actually call for personal responsibility. Perhaps Alice put her husband down several times for not putting away the dishes and called him "selfish" and "lazy." When he became sullen, she did not apologize for her choice of words; however, she continued to blame him for his depressed mood. There was no effective communication here, only assuming and blaming.

Emotional Reasoning

Emotional reasoning means using a somatic response as evidence that we have something to worry about. We use emotional reasoning when we have the butterflies in our stomach, sweaty palms, or elevated body temperature; these lead us to assume that we're anxious, fearful, or in danger. If we feel any of these visceral responses about riding in an elevator, for example, we may deduce that there is danger in riding in elevators. Another example is Alexander, a PWS, who felt tightness in his stomach before giving a presentation in class. Due to his visceral reaction, he concluded that he must be extremely nervous and that therefore he was going to stutter and mess up his speech.

Discounting the Positive

Discounting the positive means placing focus on the negatives and weaknesses, thereby dismissing the strengths and positive aspects of a situation and insisting that they "don't count." For example, Mr. Jones was improving slowly after his stroke. At first, he could not move or speak; however, with each passing day and week, he began to get out of his bed unassisted and produce most of the speech sounds intelligibly. When the speech therapist came to see him and asked how he was doing, he replied, "It's no use. I can't walk, I can't talk, and I am a shell of what I used to be." When reminded of the steady progress he had made in just a few weeks, he said it did not matter, and that he was still getting nowhere.

In another example, Jane, a perfectionist at work, always believed that she fell short, regardless of how much positive feedback she received. Jane focused on all the errors she made, on how others did a better job, and how others knew so much more than she did. She deprived herself of joy and was a drain on people whenever she voiced her bleak self-perception.

As we work on our self-awareness and understanding of our own thinking traps, we gain insight to the thinking traps of others. As a result, with compassion and sensitivity, we may teach our clients about their thinking traps and how to deal with them. We may assist them to apply this new knowledge so that they are better able to manage their behaviors and reactions.

Ask Yourself

Paying attention to thinking traps helps us gain perspective on challenging situations. Sometimes we employ more than one thinking trap at a time. Identify one or more of the five thinking traps (*jumping to conclusions* by mind-reading or fortune-telling, *overgeneralization, personalization and blame, emotional reasoning,* and *discounting the positive* for the following events:

1. A college professor with a hyperfunctional voice disorder (vocal hoarseness due to inefficient use and overuse of the voice, which may result in benign irritation or

growths on the vocal folds) has become frustrated with his difficulty maintaining appropriate vocal intensity (loudness) for the duration of his lecture.

He expresses to his speech-language pathologist that he is concerned that the class never enjoys his lectures because it is so difficult to hear him. He worries that he'll lose his job, even though he's an excellent professor who has received high praise from both students and peers. He worries that once he loses this job, he won't find another one because his voice is getting worse. As a matter of fact, everything related to his job is going poorly at this point.

Thinking Trap(s):_____

2. A middle-school student named Joe who's struggling with attention-deficit/hyperactivity disorder feels depressed. His thoughts focus on his difficulties with making friends and being part of a peer group. Although he's gotten close with several new students this year, he says that no one likes him and he may as well give up on trying to establish new relationships.

   Joe believes that he does have one good friend, who recently got in trouble in school because when he turned around to talk to Joe, the teacher noticed and punished him. Joe feels certain that he is to blame and worried that he will lose this friendship

Thinking Trap(s):_____

3. A PWS named Sam wanted to ask a girl named Samantha on a date. He approached Samantha, but when he began to address her, she waved to a friend walking by. Sam thought, "She is trying to avoid me. She does not want to go out with me. No one ever wants to go out with me."

Thinking Trap(s):_____

In *Atlas Shrugged*, Ayn Rand (1956) advised:

> Do not let your fire go out, spark by irreplaceable spark. In the hopeless swamp of the not quite, the not yet, and the not at all, do not let the hero in your soul perish and leave only frustration for the life you deserved, but have never been able to reach. The world you desire can be won, it exists, it is real, it is possible, it is yours.

Do not allow your inner critic to overpower your true inner voice or the voices of your clients and of their families.

KEY CONCEPTS

- The three obstacles—judgments, expectations, and the inner critic—steer us away from transformation and growth.
- We all judge both ourselves and others; likewise, others judge us.
- The problem is not in the judging but in the way we treat ourselves and others.
- Judgment interferes with seeing and hearing people. It shuts down communication. It alters our perspective.
- Self-awareness is key to controlling and redirecting judgments, which leads to effective communication.
- Curiosity is an antidote to judgment.

- It is essential to come to some understanding of the roots of our judgments.
- Clinicians frequently judge parents when parents experience loss, anger, fear, and denial, and when parents do not follow recommendations and resist acceptance of the process.
- There is a distinct difference between judgment and evaluation. Evaluation denotes objectivity, whereas judgment implies subjectivity.
- Collaborative partnership and trust require keeping our judgments in check and building compassion and support.
- Although expectations may occasionally be motivators, they frequently interfere with communication and foster disappointment.
- Realistic expectations are achievable and within reason.
- Unrealistic expectations are unachievable and removed from reality.
- Disappointments gain power, in part, because they are layered on previous ones (stack attack).
- Maintaining your sense of humor is crucial to keeping expectations in check.
- We must learn to hear the expectations of others without becoming defensive.
- It is crucial to hear and listen to parents' expectations even if those expectations are unrealistic.
- Our job is to clarify what is possible step-by-step and to be realistic with parents.
- When we keep expectations realistic, we leave room for our growth and for the growth of our clients.
- Maintaining personal boundaries empowers us to prevent overwhelming and unrealistic expectations.
- The inner critic or saboteur lives within all of us.
- The inner critic and our relationship with it influence how we perceive and react to situations and other individuals, as well as how we rally from adversity.
- The inner critic develops when we are very young as an outgrowth of the warnings of the adults in our lives (e.g., "Be careful," "Don't hurt yourself," "Be realistic").
- These warnings are internalized and develop as we grow, cautioning us to stay in our comfort zone.
- Negative self-image becomes a self-fulfilling prophecy.
- It is only when we become aware and accept the critic that we can be who we truly are.
- It's common to confuse the inner critic with our true inner voice; we need to distinguish between the two.
- We may experience discomfort in response to inconsistency between our core beliefs (our deep-seated view of ourselves) and what happens in our lives.
- That particular discomfort may lead a person to self-sabotage.
- Another way the inner critic may manifest is in the form of thinking traps.
- Thinking traps are entanglements in a behavior that do not serve us well.

- Thinking traps discussed in this chapter include the following:
  - Jumping to conclusions (catastrophizing): mind-reading and fortune-telling
  - Overgeneralization: a form of all-or-nothing thinking
  - Personalization and blame
  - Emotional reasoning
  - Discounting the positive
- This transformational path requires patience with the process of controlling these obstacles and is essential for our personal growth and for the growth of our clients and their families.

REFERENCES

Andersen, H. C. (1844/1983). The snow queen. In E. C. Haugaard (Trans.), *The complete fairy tales and stories*. New York, NY: Anchor Books.

Ben-Shahar, T. (2010). *Foundations of positive psychology* [PowerPoint slides]. Retrieved from www.slideshare.net/dadalaolang/1504-01intro?ref=http://positivepsychologyprogram.com/harvard-positive-psychology-course

Branden. N. (1995). *The six pillars of self-esteem: The definitive work on self-esteem by the leading pioneer in the field*. New York, NY: Bantam Books.

Brody, J. (2015, July 21). Exercise for the immediate satisfaction. *New York Times*, pp. D7.

Bronson, P., & Merryman, A. (2009). *Nurture shock*. New York, NY: Hachette Book Group.

Buckingham, M., & Clifton, D. O. (2001). *Now, discover your strengths*. New York, NY: Simon & Schuster.

Burns, D. D. (1999). *The feeling good handbook*. New York, NY: Plume.

Cameron, J. (2002). *The artist's way*. Westminster, United Kingdom: Penguin Books.

Carey, W. B., & McDevitt, S. C. (1995). *Coping with children's temperament: A guide for professionals*. New York, NY: Basic Books.

Carlson, R. (1997). *Don't sweat the small stuff and it's all small stuff: Simple ways to keep the little things from taking over your life*. New York, NY: Hyperion Books.

Cawsey, T., & Deszca, G. (2011). *Organizational change: An action oriented toolkit* (2nd ed.). Los Angeles, CA: Sage.

Covey, S. (1989). *The seven habits of highly effective people*. New York, New York: Simon & Schuster.

Faber, A., & Mazlish, E. (2005). *How to talk so teens will listen & listen so teens will talk*. New York, NY: HarperCollins.

Faber, A., & Mazlish, E. (2012). *How to talk so kids will listen & listen so kids will talk*. New York, NY: Simon & Schuster.

Firestone, R. W., Firestone, L., & Catlett, J. (2002). *Conquer your critical inner voice: A revolutionary program to counter negative thoughts and live free from imagined limitations*. Oakland, CA: New Harbinger.

Flasher, L., & Fogle, P. (2012). *Counseling skills for speech-language pathologists and audiologists*. Clifton Park, NY: Delmar Cengage Learning.

Griffith, B. A., & Frieden, G. (2000). Facilitating reflective thinking in counselor education. *Counselor Education and Supervision, 40*(2), 82–93.

Haynes, W. O., & Pindzola, R. H. (2011). *Diagnosis and evaluation in speech pathology*. New York, NY: Pearson Higher Education.

Heifetz, R. A., Grashow, A., & Linsky, M. (2009). *The practice of adaptive leadership: Tools and tactics for changing your organization and the world*. Boston, MA: Harvard Business Press.

Hoag, J. (2015). NLP perceptual positions, by John David Hoag. *Nlpls.com*. Retrieved from www.nlpls.com/articles/perceptualPositions.php

Kimsey-House, H., Kimsey-House, K., Sandahl, P., & Whitworth, L. (2011). *Co-active coaching: Changing business, transforming lives*. Boston, MA: Nicholas Brealey.

Kingsley, E. P. (1987) *Welcome to Holland*. Retrieved from www.child-autism-parent-cafe.com/welcome-to-holland.html

Luterman, D. (2008). *Counseling persons with communication disorders and their families* (5th ed.). Austin, TX: Pro-Ed.

Manolson, A., Ward, B., & Dodington, N. (1995). *You make the difference in helping your child learn*. Ontario, Canada: The Hanen Centre.

Miller, D. (2011). *A million miles in a thousand years: How I learned to live a better story*. Nashville, TN: Thomas Nelson.

Rand, A. (1956). *Atlas shrugged*. New York, NY: Penguin Group.

Reivich, K., & Shatté, A. (2002). *The resilience factor: 7 essential skills for overcoming life's inevitable obstacles.* New York, NY: Broadway Books.

Riley, J. (2002). Counseling: An approach for speech-language pathologists. *Contemporary Issues in Communication Science and Disorders, 29,* 6–16.

Sapey, B. J., & Oliver, M. (2006). *Social work with disabled people.* London, United Kingdom: Palgrave Macmillan.

Stone, H., & Stone, S. (1989). *Embracing each other.* Albion, CA: Delos.

Stone, H., & Stone, S. (1993). *Embracing your inner critic.* San Francisco, CA: Harper One.

Whitworth, L. (2007). *Co-Active Coaching: New skills for coaching people toward success in work and life.* Mountain View, CA: Davies-Black.

10

The Clinical Interview and Concluding Remarks on Change

We shall not cease from exploration/And the end of all our exploring/Will be to arrive where we started/And know the place for the first time.

—T. S. Elliot, 1943

LEARNER OUTCOMES

After reading this chapter the reader will be able to:

1. Cite and describe the elements involved in conducting a clinical interview.

2. Draw and/or describe the funnel in the post-evaluation conference.

3. Identify the five key ingredients to making change.

4. Describe the aspects of procrastination and the 5-minute rule (Ben-Shahar, 2010).

Since the diagnostic interview is the first opportunity a speech-language pathologist or audiologist has to meet with parents, children, or adult clients, the interview will also be the first opportunity to apply the lessons learned in this book. The following tools will help unify the concepts we have discussed.

THE CLINICAL INTERVIEW (THE CLINICIAN'S TOOL KIT)

It is essential that the examiner be alert for and incorporate the information gained in the client/family interview with clinical assessment results.

The clinician should pay attention to the following:

- Possible missing links in the diagnostic puzzle.

- Be aware of client and family priorities, goals, and the reasons for their goals.

Stein-Rubin, C., & Adler, B. T. *Counseling in Communication Disorders: Facilitating the Therapeutic Rehabilitation* (pp 167-179).
© 2017 Taylor & Francis Group.

- Be alert for inconsistencies in client and family information in:
  - Reports between each other's accounts.
  - Incongruities between their oral reports and clinical data.

Moreover, the clinician must note this conflicting information in the diagnostic report. To assist us in using a coaching approach during the clinical interview, we have included a list and description of coaching/counseling tools in the following section. The following toolkit will be helpful in the clinical interview and counseling process.

- Reflecting/clarifying
- Summary probe
- Clearing
- Powerful questions
- Meta-view
- Reframing
- Acknowledging

Reflecting/Clarifying

In *reflecting*, we simply mirror back to the client what she has just said. In this way, we as clinicians act as giant mirrors, and the client sees or hears herself more clearly. It is striking what evolves from simply letting the individual hear her own words. This gives the client greater access to her emotions and leads to client resourcefulness (Shirk, 2008). There are often revelations that appear for the client from this simple act. This act of reflecting also involves paraphrasing and interpreting the client's statement in our own words. Reflecting and clarifying are generally more effective than simply repeating back what the client has said. The following is an example:

> **Client:** There are so many things to do and work on; I have schools to investigate, and I'm so tired.

> **Interviewer:** It sounds like you feel overwhelmed.

As noted in Chapter 5, check in with the client when reflecting back or clarifying what has been heard, and be sure that she agrees with the paraphrase. Checking in further facilitates communication. If the client corrects or disagrees, that serves as valuable feedback, because it allows us a more representative picture about what she is feeling. Furthermore, if a client corrects reflection, this becomes an opportunity for her to clarify her own thoughts, deepen her self-discovery, and is an invitation for us to proceed. Below are two possible dialogues that may result from checking in with the client. They illustrate how a quick confirmation from her contributes to verifying the interpretation of her feelings.

> **Interviewer:** Is that true?

> **Client:** Yes, that's exactly how I feel; very overwhelmed.

> **Interviewer:** Is that true?

> **Client:** Not really overwhelmed, more afraid than overwhelmed, scared.

Summary Probe

Summary probe is often a helpful transitional device to summarize, in one's own words, what the client has told us. This is often a tactful way to consolidate or steer the conversation back on track. It also provides the opportunity to use the client's thoughts to segue into the next topic. Furthermore, the summary probe reinforces the depth of one's listening, which also ensures one has all the information in the correct sequence. Summing up the client's remarks also provides opportunity for more sharing and makes the client feel truly heard (Manning, 2009). The following is an example:

> **Clinician:** Let me just back track for a minute here to be sure that I understand: You said that your child stuttered from about the age of 3 years and became self-conscious about it this year in kindergarten? Is that right? Tell me more about that.

Clearing

Often people need to release their emotions (e.g., sadness, frustration, anger). Allow them some time to tell their stories, feel sorry for themselves, and release their negative emotions. We must use our intuition to determine an individual's pressing need to vent and express her reactions to being unfairly targeted, feeling trapped, angry, frightened, and overwhelmed. Oftentimes, once an individual releases the emotion, she is more emotionally and cognitively ready to receive information (Whitworth, 2007).

Powerful Questions

Powerful questions are open-ended, curious, introspective, and thought provoking questions. These inquiries prompt an individual to look deep inside and search for an authentic response. Do not be surprised if there is a silent pause following a powerful question. These are not the type of inquiries that people are accustomed to answering and often may require a deeper reflection. Try to limit the use of closed-ended, yes/no, or *leading questions*. When inquiries are leading they have an underlying agenda of manipulating the client toward a particular type of response. Take care to preserve and not hijack the client's agenda (Whitworth, 2007). The following are some examples of curious powerful questions:

- What do you truly want?
- How will you know you received it?
- What about that is important to you?
- What's next?
- What else?
- What would that look like?
- What does "stuck" feel like?
- What will finishing that give you?
- How would it look if your life were balanced?
- What did you learn?
- What is getting in your way?

- What have you tried so far?
- What are you willing to do?
- What's working?
- What would you like to know that you don't know today?
- How does this perspective serve you?
- What would support you in accomplishing that?
- What have you done to get the job done so far?
- What is the cost?
- What is the benefit?
- What are you saying yes to?
- What are you saying no to?
- What is one more possible way of looking at this?
- How do you give your power away?

The following powerful questions illuminate and support the client's agenda and the designed alliance during the clinical interview:

- What would you like to accomplish from today's session?
- What is one important thing you are taking away today?

Meta-View

The *meta-view* assists the individual in gaining a perspective on her situation. This is another way of saying a *bird's-eye view*. It is a miniature visualization exercise where the clinician may ask the client to envision that she is taking a ride in a helicopter. Once the client is metaphorically high up in the air, ask her, "Now what do you see from here?" When we ask the client to look down and tell us what she sees now, her perspective will usually shift to a more empowered stance. We may hear the individual respond with comments such as, "All of that does not look so important anymore," or "In the scheme of things; that does not look like such a big problem."

We may also suggest envisioning a trip into the future and looking back on this difficult time to help the client gain perspective on a difficult situation or dilemma. Visualizing may help the client project that things will fall into a rhythm and place and also to help highlight her potential accomplishments (Craig & Hess, 2010).

Reframing

Reframing relates in many ways to meta-view. Like meta-view, this tool helps the client to view her problem from another perspective. While meta-view brings the client to a metaphorically different vista, reframing helps the client redefine the problem into something positive. The client's view of reality may be causing her stress. Reframing shows the client that there are various points of view offering opportunity. While there may be many perspectives that are true, reframing focuses on the fact that we always have choice. Thus, the premise is that all individuals possess the power to choose the way they view their situation.

Reframing a point of view provides the opportunity for the client to move from a position of stuck or victim into one of control. For example, helping the client alter her perspective may reduce a client's anxiety or guilt. We may offer a powerful question such as, "Your perspective is one point of view; what is another way you might look at this?" Offering these questions, may lead to a paradigm shift for the client and consequently an epiphany best described as an intuitive "A-ha."

Readiness is an important marker for timing a reframe, for any individual, and certainly for individuals with disabilities. An example of a reframe, made by a person who stutters, might be that stuttering has been an opportunity for personal growth and developing greater sensitivity to the needs of others. The reframe may also include the fact that many people who stutter have turned their limitations into a way to foster change in the lives of others with similar challenges.

Acknowledging

Please refer to Chapter 6 on language for the *Language of Acknowledgment*.

It is our hope that the previous coaching tools are useful when communicating with clients, their families and in all relationships. We suggest practicing levels II and III listening, whenever the opportunity presents itself, asking powerful questions, and acknowledging others in everyday interactions (Whitworth, 2007).

THE POST-EVALUATION TOOLKIT

One of the most anxiety provoking clinical situations for graduate students and novice speech clinicians is the post-evaluation conference. An inexperienced clinician agonizes over a myriad of issues. These issues include communicating the diagnostic results and recommendations to the parents. Often, additional factors may arise, during the evaluation, of which the family may not have been aware. For example, a child who was brought in for an articulation disorder has been found to exhibit a significant receptive and expressive linguistic disorder. Where does one begin?

We recommend the following general sequence of events in summing up the post-evaluation conference. The diagram in Figure 10-1 has been found to provide beginning clinicians with a framework that may prove to be supportive in a difficult situation. The dialogue in a post-evaluation conference may be envisioned in the configuration of a funnel as the clinician moves from discussing general to more specific information.

Figure 10-1. The Post-Evaluation Funnel.

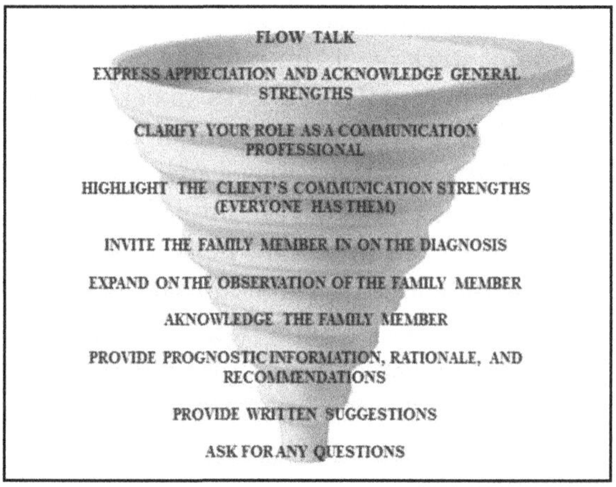

FLOW TALK

EXPRESS APPRECIATION AND ACKNOWLEDGE GENERAL
STRENGTHS

CLARIFY YOUR ROLE AS A COMMUNICATION
PROFESSIONAL

HIGHLIGHT THE CLIENT'S COMMUNICATION STRENGTHS
(EVERYONE HAS THEM)

INVITE THE FAMILY MEMBER IN ON THE DIAGNOSIS

EXPAND ON THE OBSERVATION OF THE FAMILY MEMBER

AKNOWLEDGE THE FAMILY MEMBER

PROVIDE PROGNOSTIC INFORMATION, RATIONALE, AND
RECOMMENDATIONS

PROVIDE WRITTEN SUGGESTIONS

ASK FOR ANY QUESTIONS

The following are the most important steps to include in the funnel:

- Flow talk
- Highlight general and communicative strengths
- Clarify your role
- Enlist the family in the diagnosis
- Provide written recommendations
- Question/answer period
- One important take-away

Flow Talk

Do not underestimate the power of chitchat. *Flow talk* provides a soothing and humane transition in an otherwise stressful situation. This is an important part of our professional interaction with our clients and family members (Csikszentmihalyi, 1997).

Highlight Positive Attributes

Following flow talk, the examiner moves into acknowledging the general personality and/or intellectual strengths of the client (e.g., "It was a pleasure to meet and work with Suzy today. She has a delightful sense of humor and gives everything her best effort.") After highlighting those general strengths, the clinician clarifies her role as a professional to the parent or client.

Clarify Your Role

The general public is not generally aware of the plethora of responsibilities woven into the fabric of the role of a speech-language pathology. It is important to explain that we do not simply treat a mouth. We find it helpful to relay that we are communication specialists and look at all aspects of spoken and written language. We look at numerous features of speech to include voice quality, pronunciation of sounds, and the fluent forward movement of speech.

Highlight Communication Strengths

At the previous juncture in the dialogue, the clinician may segue into the features of communication that she found to be areas of strength for this client. It is important to inform a parent that their child has communicative strengths (see Chapter 7). For example, a child may present with a receptive/expressive language delay; however, the child may also exhibit appropriate articulation, voice quality, and fluency. Furthermore, the oral peripheral examination may have been normal, exhibiting intact structures and function to support speech. One may always approach a situation from a position of strength and explain to the client and family that these positive features will serve the client well in therapy.

Enlist Family in the Diagnosis

Following illumination of the client's areas of relative strength, the clinician may want to engage the client or family in sharing or reiterating their areas of concern or perception of the client's difficulty. We prefer using the family or client's antecedents from the clinical interview and tie them into our own impressions to create a complete diagnostic description (Haynes & Pindzola, 2008). For example, "You mentioned earlier that when Jimmy relates the events of his day you cannot always follow his recount."

Approach the family members or client as naturally creative, resourceful, and whole, and as having the answers to their own questions. It is important to remember that the parent is the expert on the child's life (Luterman, 2008). In this way, we may elicit the diagnosis as well as suggestions, collaboratively. For example, at the close of the post-evaluation conference, we suggest asking the client and/or family member what they noticed during the evaluation. Their insights are often surprising. In addition, their input may alleviate the pressure on the diagnostician to have to know everything and lessen the impact of possible bad news. This collaboration maximizes client-family openness, trust, and follow through.

State what you observed about the client's areas in need of support using the family's antecedents. Discuss the general areas in need of support based on formal and informal test results. Then proceed to elaborate or move to the specific areas of difficulty. For example, a child may perform in the average range on the Test of Auditory Processing 3rd Edition in all areas, with the exception of two—auditory comprehension and reasoning. Explain the purpose of the test and clarify that performance in most of the areas was at least average with the exception of the two that were below average. The clinician might say something like, "In most of the skills that have been shown to support reading, she performed age-appropriately. She experienced difficulty in only two out of seven subtests, where listening comprehension and responding to more abstract questions were involved." Be honest and authentic without providing excessive technical detail. Follow the parent's lead in providing additional specific information.

Once we summarize the issues to be addressed in therapy, check in with the family. For example, we may want to ask the family how this feedback fits with their gut feelings. Do the analysis and recommendations resonate for them? Does the information make sense? Typically, if they have been involved in the assessment and have been acknowledged for their observations and resourcefulness, they will maintain a positive attitude and be eager to initiate a collaborative effort toward remediation. We recommend providing a *prognosis*, how likely the client is to improve with or without therapy, with an associated rationale. For example, "Suzy is a bright and motivated child. She is fortunate to have a wonderful supportive family. We anticipate that she will progress nicely in therapy."

Provide Written Recommendations

Prior to dismissing the client and family, it is advisable to provide written recommendations whether or not they are commencing therapy immediately. Aside from helping them, our suggestions empower the client and family with immediate ways to help themselves and their children. Our suggestions may mitigate our client's and/or parents' overwhelmed feelings and help give them direction. Suggestions may include specific shared book reading activities with particular books, phonemic awareness exercises such as rhyme, songs and/or finger plays, or initiating step one of a hierarchy of feared situations.

Questions and Take-Away

Offer an opportunity for questions once the recommendations have been made. In addition, ask the client or family what is one important thing she is taking away from the evaluation process. This question serves to put the finishing bow on the first encounter. This question will also stimulate and deepen the learning process and lend itself to the individual's feeling of being cared for and productive (Whitworth, 2007).

Ask Yourself

Role Play at the end of the course. One person is the evaluator or therapist, the other a parent, and the third is observer. Create a case scenario for a particular disorder. Engage in a post-evaluation conference. The observer takes notes. Do this three times so that each person plays each role.

CONCLUDING REMARKS ON CHANGE

When we first started to work on this book, we were able to visualize the final product. We had already completed a chapter in *A Guide to Clinical Assessment and Professional Report Writing in Speech-Language Pathology,* which was our first collaboration. What we didn't know was what to expect about the two of us working so closely together, for an extensive period of time, to produce a clear, cohesive, and user-friendly textbook that would articulate our common message. After all we are two strong-minded women with definitive ideas and opinions; how would we meld our thought processes to produce a product of which we would both be proud? We wondered, with uncertainty, how this entire process would play out. Would we understand each other? Would we have frequent conflicts or end up hating each other when all this was over? How would we mesh our different writing styles, schedules, moods, and stamina to achieve our ultimate goal?

The following were five key factors that we now realize influenced the completion of this daunting project:

- The first factor was our intrinsic motivation.
- Second, we were ready and willing.
- The third key factor was that we repeatedly visualized the final result.
- Fourth, we applied effort as we worked together feverishly and frequently (Ben-Shahar, 2010).
- Finally, togetherness became a dance of relationship—a metaphor for the therapeutic alliance.

We both observed ourselves instinctively, putting aside our egos and our need to be right in the interest of our project. Rather than assume the role of all-knowing experts (Oullette, 2004), we listened deeply and got genuinely curious about what the other was saying. It became far more important to really hear the other than to be "right." We gave each other space to speak thoughts and feelings aloud and to come to our own conclusions, sometimes individually, and often together. As the work unfolded, we began to work synergistically to the point we often had the same thought, at the same moment, with the identical idea to solve the problem.

As we worked, we learned from and acknowledged each other's strengths, giving us better connections with who we were and stronger self-esteem. We also mitigated each other's frustration by flipping around our negative thoughts and focusing on the strengths of our project. We got more familiar with what we were good at and how we could contribute, not only to the textbook, but professionally and in everyday life as well. We had mutual respect. We honored each other's opinions and made compromises, which seemed minor in the face of what we were trying to accomplish. We took personal responsibility for any mistakes we made, accepted each other's missteps, and granted each other and ourselves the permission to be human. Most importantly, we laughed a lot along the way and had fun co-creating and watching a labor of love flourish.

There were times when one of us needed to empathize with the way the other was feeling, whether discouraged, tired, or confused. We knew how to encourage and support each other under those circumstances, so that we could consistently move forward. We established a safe holding container of trust (Geller, 2002) and talked about real issues—personal, emotional, and sensitive. We removed our masks for each other so that we could truly see, know, and be seen and known by the other. This became the basis of our relationship.

At this point, we invite you to take a look at your own desire for change to reach a particular goal. What impassioned goal do you hope to accomplish? What is it you really want to do or to become? We suggest looking at those five ingredients for positive change. Let's examine the fifth factor, *working together,* in particular. The following are some suggestions for accomplishing the fifth aspect to positive change:

- Enlist a friend(s) to balance out your strengths, offer support, and add to the thinking process and excitement.
- Gather supports to rally around you; open up to individuals who are genuinely happy for you.
- Consider joining a group of people with a common goal.

- Free yourself from those who discourage you and mirror your saboteur. Speak your goal out loud to those positive individuals.
- Write it down and describe what difference it would make in your life.
- Write down one small step you are committed to taking.
- Give yourself a time frame.
- Make yourself accountable to your buddy.
- Watch yourself close the gap from where you are to where you want to be.
- Notice how you are already doing it.
- Acknowledge yourself—mark the goal with a celebration; do something special for yourself. Congratulations, you are on your way.

REMEMBERING AND APPLYING LESSONS LEARNED

Phillip Drucker, at the conclusion of one of his lectures, commented to his audience that at the end of the lecture he did not wish to hear how informative, dynamic, and inspiring his presentation was. He preferred to know, down the road, what his audience noticed they were doing differently (Ben-Shahar, 2010). As we look back to the lessons within this book, we realize how difficult it may be, at times, to remember how and when to apply what we have learned. Students will sometimes acknowledge this by saying, "Oh, I did learn this and forgot to apply it in this situation."

Forgetting is common for everyone, and of course, trying to remember everything at once may be overwhelming. The question for each of us to ask ourselves is, "How do we remember to stay on the path of transformation rather than entering the 'forgetting mode'?" The following strategies help us remember lessons learned:

- Accept our human qualities and know that forgetting will happen.
- We must not blame ourselves for forgetting.
- Observe, listen, and assess your communicative exchanges.
- Select one concept or tool to focus upon.
- Review the material periodically.
- Practice the material by coaching with a buddy.
- We may only be spontaneous in our counseling by developing a firm grasp and practicing the lessons within this book.

These suggestions have wide applicability for our growth as well as for the growth of our clients and their families.

Procrastination

Procrastination may interfere with progress, achievement, and change. Ben-Shahar (2010) notes that the hardest part of completing a dreaded project is getting started. He suggests the *5-minute rule*. The rule encourages a person to frame out a short manageable period of time, such as 5 minutes, to get started. If we assign ourselves only 5 minutes, to complete seemingly daunting tasks, we might tell ourselves that all we need to do is to work for 5 minutes. Once we've spent 5 minutes "doing," we've gotten through the hardest part—starting. We've broken up our task into small, manageable goals (5-minute chunks), and after a while, we tend to keep going, because we're on a roll. For example, when an individual procrastinates about exercising, she may try incorporating the 5-minute rule, and go on the treadmill for only 5 minutes. Once the individual is on the machine for 5 minutes, she is likely to want to continue. Clinically, when writing a professional report, a clinician may procrastinate initiating the task. We recommend remembering the 5-minute rule, and once 5 minutes have passed, the clinician is likely to continue writing. In the therapy room, we may engage a child in an activity for 5 minutes, and oftentimes, the child will be surprised that she was able to sustain her attention for a longer period of time (Box 10-1).

Box 10-1

A clinical example of the 5-minute rule is a behavior-modification point system used by a clinician who was working with a difficult 4-year-old boy. She engaged him in a picture card game that required him to make pairs of cards. For every 15 points he earned, he would receive a reward. After he had achieved 9 points, the boy wanted to stop, yet the clinician encouraged him to keep going since he only needed 6 more matches to get his prize. By the time he achieved the 15 points, he had become so involved in the activity that he decided not to stop until he had matched up the entire box of cards. The child not only got his reward, but he was also proud of himself for exceeding the original goal.

Ask Yourself

1. As a summary exercise for this book, read each of the following clinician responses, then write what counseling attitude, approach, and/or tool is reflected in each statement.

   a. "I'm sorry to hear that. Did anything good come out of the situation?"

   b. "Wow, that's awful. On the other hand, I'm pretty impressed with how positive you've managed to stay about the whole thing."

   c. "Ooh. How do you typically handle that?"

d. "If only [name] had the experience/wisdom/work ethic that you did!"

e. "Please, correct me if I'm wrong, but it sounds like you're upset because..."

ANSWER KEY

a. Deepening the learning and highlighting strengths
b. Empathy, acknowledgment, highlighting strengths
c. Solution-focused brief therapy (SFBT), exceptions, past behavior as evidence
d. Acknowledgment
e. Deep listening, reflecting, and summarizing
f. SFBT, focus on strengths, and on what is working

2. What's one thing you will do differently as a result of reading this book?

KEY CONCEPTS

- To arrive at a proper diagnosis, the clinician must pay attention to missing links in the diagnostic puzzle, previous reports, incongruities between all reports, and clinical data.
- The following tool kit will be helpful in the clinical interview:
  - Reflecting/clarifying
  - Summary probe
  - Clearing
  - Powerful questions
  - Meta-view
  - Reframing
  - Acknowledging
  - Using silence
  - Meeting and managing the saboteur

- The post-evaluation "funnel" includes the following:
  - Flow talk
  - Highlight general and communicative strengths
  - Clarify your role as clinician
  - Enlist the family in diagnosis
  - Written recommendations
  - Question/answer period
  - One important take-away
- The following are the five key factors for change:
  - Intrinsic motivation
  - Readiness and willingness
  - Visualizing the final result
  - Effort
  - Togetherness
- Forgetting lessons learned is common for everyone.
- Procrastination may interfere with progress, achievement, and change.
- The 5-minute rule, an antidote to procrastination, encourages a person to frame out a short manageable period of time to get started.

REFERENCES

Ben-Shahar, T. (2010). *Foundations of positive psychology* [PowerPoint slides]. Retrieved from www.slideshare.net/dadalaolang/1504-01intro?ref=http://positivepsychologyprogram.com/harvard-positive-psychology-course.

Craig, W., & Hess, R. (2010). Coach training alliance learning accelerator [CD]. Boulder, CO: Coach Training Alliance.

Csikszentmihalyi, M. (1997). *Finding flow: The psychology of engagement with everyday life.* New York, NY: Basic Books.

Eliot, T. S. (1943). Little gidding. *Columbia University.* Retrieved from www.columbia.edu/itc/history/winter/w3206/edit/tseliotlittlegidding.html.

Geller, E. (2002). A reflective model of supervision in speech-language pathology: Process and practice. *The Clinical Supervisor, 20*(2), 191–200.

Haynes, W. O., & Pindzola, R. H. (2008). *Diagnosis and evaluation in speech pathology.* (7th ed.). Boston, MA: Allyn & Bacon.

Luterman, D. (2008). *Counseling persons with communication disorders and their families* (5th ed.). Austin, TX: Pro-Ed.

Manning, W. H. (2009). Clinical decision making in fluency disorders (3rd ed.). San Diego, CA: Singular.

Ouellette, S. E. (2004). Clinical issues: Applications of solution-focused concepts to the practice of speech-language pathology. *SIG 1 Perspectives on Language Learning and Education, 11*(1), 8–14.

Shirk, A. (2008). *Foundations of the co-active approach to coaching.* Draft.

Whitworth, L. (2007). *Co-active coaching: New skills for coaching people toward success in work and life.* Mountainview, CA: Davies-Black Training Institute.

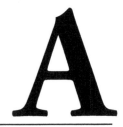

Cultural Competence Checklist

AMERICAN SPEECH-LANGUAGE-HEARING ASSOCIATION

Cultural Competence Checklist: **Personal Reflection**

This tool was developed to heighten your awareness of how you view clients/patients from culturally and linguistically diverse (CLD) populations.
*There is no answer key; however, you should review responses that you rated 5, 4, and even 3.

Ratings:
1 Strongly Agree
2 Agree
3 Neutral
4 Disagree
5 Strongly Disagree

____ I treat all of my clients with respect for their culture.

____ I do not impose my beliefs and value systems on my clients, their family members, or their friends.

____ I believe that it is acceptable to use a language other than English in the U.S.

____ I accept my clients' decisions as to the degree to which they choose to acculturate into the dominant culture.

____ I provide services to clients who are GLBTQ (Gay, Lesbian, Bisexual, Transgender, or Questioning).

____ I am driven to respond to others' insensitive comments or behaviors.

____ I do not participate in insensitive comments or behaviors.

____ I am aware that the roles of family members may differ within or across culture or families.

____ I recognize family members and other designees as decision makers for services and support.

____ I respect non-traditional family structures (e.g., divorced parents, same gender parents, grandparents as caretakers).

____ I understand the difference between a communication disability and a communication difference.

____ I understand that views of the aging process may influence the clients'/families' decision to seek intervention.

____ I understand that there are several American English dialects. I recognize that all English speakers use a dialect of English.

I understand that the use of a foreign accent or limited English skill is not a reflection of:

____ Reduced intellectual capacity

____ The ability to communicate clearly and effectively in a native language

I understand how culture can affect child-rearing practices such as:

____ Discipline

____ Dressing

____ Toileting

____ Feeding

____ Self-help skills

____ Expectations for the future

____ Communication

I understand the impact of culture on life activities, such as:

____ Education

____ Family roles

____ Religion/faith-based practices

____ Gender roles

____ Alternative medicine

____ Customs or superstitions

____ Employment

____ Perception of time

____ Views of wellness

____ Views of disabilities

____ The value of Western medical treatment

I understand my clients' cultural norms may influence communication in many ways, including:

____ Eye contact

____ Interpersonal space

____ Use of gestures

____ Comfort with silence

____ Turn-taking

____ Topics of conversation

____ Asking and responding to questions

____ Greetings

____ Interruptions

____ Use of humor

____ Decision-making roles

*While several sources were consulted in the development of this checklist, the following document inspired its design:
Goode, T. D. (1989, revised 2002). Promoting cultural and linguistic competence self-assessment checklist for personnel Providing services and supports in early intervention and childhood settings.

Reference this material as: American Speech-Language-Hearing Association. (2010). *Cultural Competence Checklist: Personal reflection.* Available from www.asha.org/uploadedFiles/practice/multicultural/personalreflections.pdf.

Stein-Rubin, C., & Adler, B. T. *Counseling in Communication Disorders: Facilitating the Therapeutic Rehabilitation* (p 181). © 2017 Taylor & Francis Group.

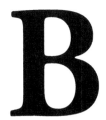

Suggested Readings

Albom, M. (1997). *Tuesdays with Morrie: An old man, a young man, and life's greatest lesson.* New York, NY: Broadway.

Albom, M. (2003). *The five people you meet in Heaven.* New York, NY: Hyperion.

Albom, M. (2006). *For one more day.* New York, NY: Hyperion.

Axline, V. (1967). *Dibs in search of self.* New York, NY: Ballantine.

Barron, J. (2002). *There's a boy in here.* Arlington, TX: Future Horizons.

Beattie, M. (1992). *Codependent no more: How to stop controlling others and start caring for yourself.* Center City, MN: Hazelden.

Ben-Shahar, T. (2007). *Happier: Learn the secrets to daily joy and lasting fulfillment.* New York, NY: McGraw Hill.

Boone, D. (2009). *Damn shoes and other talking tales: A selection of true narratives about people who directly and indirectly experience communication disorders.* Tucson, AZ: Forman.

Branden, N. (1994). *The six pillars of self-esteem.* New York, NY: Bantam.

Breathnach, S. (1995). *Simple abundance: A daybook of comfort and joy.* New York, NY: Warner.

Briggs, D. (1986). *Celebrate your self: Enhancing your self-esteem.* New York, NY: Broadway.

Brown, B. (2012). *Daring greatly: How the courage to be vulnerable transforms the way we live, love, parent, and lead.* New York, NY: Gotham Books.

Buchman, D. (2006). *A special education: One family's journey through the maze of learning disabilities.* Cambridge, MA: Da Capo Lifelong.

Burns, D. (2006). *Panic attacks: The new, drug-free anxiety therapy that can change your life.* New York, NY: Morgan Road Books.

Cameron, J. (2002). *The artist's way: A spiritual path to higher creativity.* New York, NY: Tarcher/Putnam.

Carlson, R. (1997). *Don't sweat the small stuff...and it's all small stuff.* New York, NY: Hyperion.

Carson, R. (2003). *Taming your gremlin.* New York, NY: HarperCollins.

Chopra, D. (1997). *The seven spiritual laws of success for parents.* New York, NY: Harmony.

Clifton, D., & Anderson, E. (2006). *Strengths quest: Discover and develop your strengths in academics, career, and beyond.* New York, NY: Gallup Press.

Cousins, N. (2005). *Anatomy of an illness as perceived by the patient.* New York, NY: W.W. Norton.

Covey, S. R. (1989). *The seven habits of highly effective people.* New York, NY: Simon and Schuster.

Covey, S. R., Merrill, R., & Merrill, R. (1994). *First things first.* New York, NY: Fireside.

Crum, T. (2006). *Three deep breaths: Finding power and purpose in a stressed-out world.* Oakland, CA: Berrett-Koehler Publishers, Inc.

Daloz, L. (1999). *Mentor: Guiding the journey of adult learners.* San Francisco, CA: Jossey-Bass.

Davich, V. (2004). *8 minute meditation.* New York, NY: Penguin Books.

de Shazer, S. (1985). *Keys to solution in brief therapy.* New York, NY: W.W. Norton.

Diener, E., & Diener, R. (2008). *Happiness: Unlocking the mysteries of psychological wealth.* Malden, MA: Blackwell Publishing.

Dyer, W. (1989). *You'll see it when you believe it: The way to your personal transformation.* New York, NY: Quill (HarperCollins).

Dyer, W. (2001). *10 secrets for success and inner peace.* Carlsbad, CA: Hay House.

Edwards, K. (2006). *The memory keeper's daughter.* New York, NY: Penguin.

Faber, A., & Mazlish, E. (1996). *How to talk so kids can learn at home and in school.* New York, NY: Simon and Schuster.

Fisher, R., & Ury, W. (2011). *Getting to yes: Negotiating agreement without giving in.* New York, NY: Penguin.

Fredrickson, B. (2009). *Positivity: Top-notch research reveals 3 to 1 ratio that will change your life.* New York, NY: Three Rivers Press.

Grandin, T. (2006). *Thinking in pictures and other reports from my life with autism.* New York, NY: Vintage.

Grealy, L. (2003). *Autobiography of a face.* New York, NY: Perennial.

Greenberger, D., & Padesky, C. (1995). *Mind over mood: Change how you feel by changing the way you think.* New York, NY: The Guilford Press.

Hallowell, E. (1996). *When you worry about the child you love: Emotional and learning problems in children.* New York, NY: Simon & Schuster.

Hampshire, S. (1982). *Susan's story: An autobiographical account of my struggle with dyslexia.* New York, NY: St. Martin's Press.

Hampshire, S. (1990). *Susan's story: An autobiographical account of my struggle with words.* London, United Kingdom: Sidgwick & Jackson.

Hay, L. (2004). *You can heal your life.* Carlsbad, CA: Hay House.

Hay, L. (2013). *All is well: Heal your body with medicine, affirmations, and intuition.* Carlsbad, CA: Hay House.

Heath, C., & Heath, D. (2010). *Switch: How to change things when change is hard.* New York, NY: Broadway.

Helmsetter, S. (1982). *What to say when you talk to yourself.* New York, NY: Pocket Books.

Hyman, B., & Pedrick, C. (2010). *The OCD workbook: Your guide to breaking free from obsessive-compulsive disorder.* Oakland, CA: New Harbinger Publications.

Ivey, A., Ivey, M., & Zalaquatt, C. (2010). *Intentional interviewing & counseling: Facilitating client development in a multicultural society.* Belmont, CA: Brooks/Cole, Cengage Learning.

James, J., Friedman, R., & Matthew, L. L. (2001). *When children grieve: For adults to help children deal with death, divorce, pet loss, moving and other losses.* New York, NY: Quill.

Jeffers, S. (1987). *Feel the fear...and do it anyway.* New York, NY: Random House.

Kashdan, T. (2009). *Curious? Discover the missing ingredient to a fulfilling life.* New York, NY: Harper Collins.

Kegan, R., & Lahey, L. (2001). *How the way we talk can change the way we work: Seven languages for transformation.* San Francisco, CA: Jossey-Bass.

Kegan, R., & Lahey, L. (2009). *Immunity to change: How to overcome it and unlock the potential in yourself and your organization (leadership for the common good).* Boston, MA: Harvard Business Press.

Kimsey-House, H., Kimsey-House, K., Sandahl, P., & Whitworth, L. (2008). *Co-active coaching: Changing business transforming lives: The book that helped define the field of professional coaching.* Boston, MA: Nicholas Brealey Publishing.

Lama XIV, D. (1999). *The art of happiness : A handbook for living.* New York, NY: Riverhead

Langer, E. (1989). *Mindfulness.* Boston, MA: Da Capo Press.

Lerner, H. (1989). *The dance of intimacy: A woman's guide to courageous acts of change in key relationships.* New York, NY: Harper & Row.

Lerner, H. (2001). *The mother dance: How children change your life.* New York, NY: Harper/Quill.

Lerner, H. (2005). *The dance of anger: A woman's guide to changing the patterns of intimate relationships.* New York, NY: Perennial Currents.

Loeher, J., & Schwartz, T. (2003). *The power of full engagement.* New York, NY: Simon and Schuster.

Lyubomirsky, S. (2007). *The how of happiness: A scientific approach to getting the life you want.* New York, NY: Penguin Press.

Mackenzie, R. (2001). *Setting limits with your strong willed child.* New York, NY: Three Rivers Press.

Miller, W., & Rollnick, S. (2013) *Motivational interviewing: Preparing people for change.* New York, NY: The Guilford Press.

Newman, M., & Berkowitz, B. (1971). *How to be your own best friend.* New York, NY: Ballantine.

O'Connor, J., & Lages, A. (2004). *Coaching with NLP: How to be a master coach.* London, United Kingdom: Element.

Padesky, C., & Greenberger, D. (1995). *Clinician's guide to mind over mood.* New York, NY: The Guilford Press.

Palacio, R. J. (2012). *Wonder.* New York, NY: Random House.

Patterson, G. R. (1977). *Living with children: New methods for parents & teachers.* Champaign, IL: Research Press.

Pausch, R. (2008). *The last lecture.* New York, NY: Hyperion.

Peck, M. S. (1978). *The road less travelled: A new psychology of love, traditional values and spiritual growth.* New York, NY: Touchstone.

Phelau, T. (2003). *1-2-3 magic: Effective discipline for children 2-12.* Glen Ellyn, IL: Parent Magic Inc.

Powell, J. (1989). *Happiness is an inside job.* Allen, TX: Tabor.

Rath, T., & Harte, J. (2010). *Wellbeing: The five essential elements.* New York, NY: Gallup Press.

Reivich, K., & Shatté, A. (2002). *The resilience factor: 7 keys to finding your inner strength and overcoming life's hurdles.* New York, NY: Broadway Books.

Ruiz, M. (1997). *The four agreements: A practical guide to personal freedom a toltec wisdom book.* San Rafael, CA: Amber-Allen.

Saleeby, D. (1992). *The strengths perspective in social work practice.* New York, NY: Longman Pub. Group.

Sanford, J. (1982). *Between people—Communicating one to one*. Mahwah, NJ: Paulist Press

Schroff, L., & Tresniowski, A. (2011). *An invisible thread: The true story of an 11-year-old panhandler, a busy sales executive, and an unlikely meeting with destiny*. New York, NY: Howard.

Seigel, B. (1986). *Love, medicine & miracles: Lessons learned about self-healing from a surgeon's experience with exceptional patients*. New York, NY: Harper & Row.

Seigel, B. (1989). *Peace, love and healing: Bodymind communications & the path to self-healing: An exploration*. New York, NY: Harper & Row.

Seligman, M. E. P. (2002). *Authentic happiness: Using the new positive psychology to realize your potential for lasting fulfillment*. New York, NY: Atria.

Shafir, R. (2003). *The zen of listening: Mindful communication in the age of distraction*. Wheaton, IL: Quest.

Stein-Rubin, C., & Fabus, R. (2012). *A guide to clinical assessment and professional report writing in speech-language pathology*. Clifton Park, NY: Delmar/Cengage Learning.

Stiffelman, S. (2012). *Parenting without power struggles: Raising joyful, resilient kids while staying cool, calm, and connected*. New York, NY: Atria.

Stone, D. (1999). *Embracing ourselves: The voice of dialogue manual*. Novato, CA: Nataraj.

Tannen, D. (2006). *You're wearing that?: Understanding mothers & daughters in conversation*. New York, NY: Ballantine.

Tolle, E. (1999). *The power of now: A guide to spiritual enlightenment*. Novato, CA: New World Library.

Zander, R., & Zander, B. (2000). *The art of possibility: Transforming professional and personal life*. Boston, MA: Harvard Business School Press.

Index

Printed in the United States
by Baker & Taylor Publisher Services